Surgery:
Review for New National Boards

Surgery:
Review for New National Boards

Glenn W. Geelhoed, M.D., M.P.H., F.A.C.S.
Professor of Surgery
Professor of International Medical Education
George Washington University Medical Center
Washington, D.C.

J&S

J&S Publishing Company Inc., Alexandria, Virginia

J&S

Composition and Layout: Ronald C. Bohn, Ph. D.
Cover Design and Editing: Kurt E. Johnson, Ph. D.
Printing Supervisor: Robert Perotti, Jr.
Printing: Goodway Graphics, Springfield, Virginia

Library of Congress Catalog Card Number 94-079792

ISBN 0-9632873-5-4

© 1995 by J & S Publishing Company, Inc., Alexandria, Virginia

Printed in the United States of America. All rights reserved. Except as permitted under the Copyright Act of 1976, no part of this publication may be reproduced or distributed in any form or by any means or stored in a data base or retrieval system, without the prior written permission of the publisher.

10 9 8 7 6 5 4 3 2 1

Dedication

The author would like to dedicate this book to Timothy S. Harrison, M.D., Professor of Surgery and Physiology, Milton S. Hershey Medical Center. Dr. Harrison has been a role model as surgeon, endocrinologic investigator, teacher and internationalist. I have enjoyed combined surgical educational efforts in Ann Arbor, Hershey, Boston, and our "surgical explorations" in Pakistan, Africa, Oman and the Arabian Gulf.

Table of Contents

Preface .... *vii*

Acknowledgements .... *viii*

Chapter I   *Surgical Principles and Patient Management* *1*

Chapter II   *Abdominal Surgery* *49*

Chapter III   *Cardiovascular and Thoracic Surgery* *105*

Chapter IV   *Emergency and Trauma Surgery* *131*

Chapter V   *Head and Neck Surgery; Endocrine Surgery* *157*

Chapter VI   *Urogenital Surgery; Breast Surgery* *187*

Chapter VII   *Neurosurgery; Pediatric Surgery; Orthopedic Surgery* *219*

Preface

This book is designed to enable you to review in just 1-2 days all of the basic surgical sciences you studied in medical school. I have been able to condense a review of the clinical surgical sciences into a single book because of the new format of the National Board Part II Examination. It is no longer prudent to review exhaustively the clinical science courses because the new examination format no longer rewards an encyclopedic knowledge of the clinical sciences. Instead, the new examinations test knowledge of the scientific basis of disease and the ability to apply clinical scientific information to the clinical reasoning process. Consequently, the most efficient way to study for the new exam is 1) to review only the most clinically relevant material from each clinical science course and 2) to focus on the application of this material to the solution of clinical problems. These two new study features form the core of this text.

If you answer every question and read all the tutorials in this book, you can cover within 2 days all of the most clinically relevant information from your surgical science courses. You will find that many surgical facts reviewed or learned anew will be presented in the context of a surgical case or an illustration. We hope that the clinical cases and illustrations will enhance your understanding, recall and application of the information. Finally, you will learn from the tutorials how surgical information is used by knowledgeable physicians to understand the courses of diseases and the significance of abnormal findings.

Glenn W. Geelhoed, M.D., M.P.H., F.A.C.S.
Washington, D.C.
November, 1994

Acknowledgements

The author would like to thank Dr. Ronald C. Bohn for his expertise in formatting these documents for production. He would also like to thank Diane C. Downing, R.N., M.P.H. for preparing the typescript. The author is grateful for all of this help and acknowledges any errors in this book as his own.

Disclaimer

The clinical information presented in this book is accurate for the purposes of review for licensure examinations but in no way should be used to treat patients or substituted for modern clinical training. Proper diagnosis and treatment of patients requires comprehensive evaluation of all symptoms, careful monitoring for adverse responses to treatment and assessment of the long-term consequences of therapeutic intervention.

Figure Credits

The illustrations used in this book are taken from the author's personal collection.

CHAPTER I
SURGICAL PRINCIPLES AND PATIENT MANAGEMENT

Items 1-4

  (A) Hypovolemic shock
  (B) Septic shock
  (C) Both
  (D) Neither

1. renal impairment

2. cold, pale, constricted extremities

3. treated with high volume infusion

4. increased cardiac output

Items 5-8

  (A) Wound healing by primary intention
  (B) Wound healing by secondary intention
  (C) Both
  (D) Neither

5. less scarring

6. contraction is prominent

7. inflammation is involved in the process

8. accelerated by steroids

ANSWERS AND TUTORIAL ON ITEMS 1-4

The answers are: **1-C; 2-A; 3-C; 4-B**.

Hypovolemic and septic shock are both types of inadequate nutrient flow, and the one sensitive vascular perfusion bed that recognizes this and loses function is the kidney. In both forms of shock, the kidneys are a sensitive indicator of shock. The classic signs of increased vasoconstriction in the periphery, in order to preserve the decreased volume for circulation through the core, are classically apparent in hypovolemic shock. However, warm, pink and well-perfused extremities and nail beds are evident in septic shock, since in this instance the cardiac output is increased. The increased cardiac output is principally a function of decreased peripheral vascular resistance, but there would be a relative insufficiency of nutrient flow to the core because of this shunting. Therefore, both hypovolemic shock and septic shock are treated with high volume infusion. It is sometimes difficult for the observer to appreciate that a patient with warm extremities and a bounding pulse is in shock, but cerebral function, renal output, and an impending acidosis reflect that this is a status of anaerobic tissue metabolism, and that whatever flow is being delivered is not adequately sustaining aerobic metabolism.

ANSWERS AND TUTORIAL ON ITEMS 5-8

The answers are: **5-A; 6-B; 7-C; 8-D**.

A wound is an injury that resolves through inflammation, so wound healing by either intention involves inflammatory processes. If that inflammation is controlled, and if linear apposition of the tissue to be scarred is made surgically contiguous, there is less scarring, which is what the intent of primary intention wound healing is. Wound healing by second intention occurs if a tissue defect is left that must be filled from the lateral sides, not only by re-epithelialization possible directly, but by granulation before epithelial overgrowth can cover the granulation. This takes longer, producing more scarring. Contraction is a prominent process as granulation precedes epithelialization, and the resultant closure is smaller than the original wound which has shrunk over the course of that progress.

There are any number of things that can interfere with the resolution of the inflammatory process and a healed wound, but few things that accelerate it, and none of them that can improve over the basic process of primary intention healing. Chief among the inhibitors of wound healing is infection, but foreign body reaction, tension and mobility, and some drugs are prominent as well. Corticosteroids, being anti-inflammatory, actually inhibit the healing process rather than contribute to it, and that is true for both primary and secondary intention healing.

Items 9-12

(A) Resectability
(B) Operability
(C) Both
(D) Neither

9. sometimes improved by radiotherapy

10. contraindication criteria for operation

11. most dependent on host factors

12. determines that operation *should* be done

Items 13-16

(A) Hypercalcemia
(B) Hypocalcemia
(C) Both
(D) Neither

13. tetany

14. cardiac systolic arrest

15. cardiac hyperirritability arrhythmia

16. acidosis improves

ANSWERS AND TUTORIAL ON ITEMS 9-12

The answers are: **9-A; 10-C; 11-B; 12-D**.

Operability is a function of the patient's condition, and resectability is a feature of the extent of the tumor and the surgical skill and equipment at hand. Either/and/or both of these features are criteria for contraindicating operation. For example, a resectable tumor in an inoperable patient or an unresectable tumor in an operable patient both are contraindications for proceeding. Occasionally radiotherapy and more rarely chemotherapy can convert resectability if the margins of the tumor are brought away from vital organs, for example. By the same token, a patient may be inoperable but after a period of "buffing" through use of cardiotonic agents, nutritional support, and conditioning, the patient operability may have improved, and — it is hoped — the resectability of the tumor has not changed.

That a patient is operable and the tumor resectable do not automatically indicate operation, since neither determines that an operation *should* be done. Such an example is a prostate cancer limited to the confines of one lobe in an otherwise healthy 95 year-old man. Factors that go into clinical judgment as to whether a tumor should be resected when it is agreed that it can be in a patient who can tolerate the operation should extend to whether direct benefit will outweigh the risk, discomfort, cost and time invested in this imperfect process. If the tumor just mentioned, for example, is not giving debilitating obstruction or threatened loss of productive life expectancy, the very presence of the tumor and willingness of the patient to undergo a treatment that can be performed with anticipated success does not mean that the operation should proceed. Clinical judgment, therefore, must include tumor resectability and patient operability, each of which are factors necessary, but not sufficient, for recommendation of operation.

ANSWERS AND TUTORIAL ON ITEMS 13-16

The answers are: **13-B; 14-A; 15-B; 16-B**.

Ionized calcium is a very important component of extracellular fluid and is carefully maintained at a level and ionized state through buffering and disassociation from readily available reserves. Since it is one of the most zealously guarded elements in the body with respect to a narrow range in which its biologic functions are optimum, disorders on either side give considerable symptoms and compensatory efforts toward correction. Hypocalcemia gives irritability and lower threshold for excitation in both neural and muscular conduction and contraction. This is noted by the patient with distressing symptoms of tetany, and the clinician worries about the cardiac arrhythmias that are also reflections of this hyperexcitability.

Because hydrogen ion and calcium compete for binding sites on serum albumin, an increase in hydrogen ion concentration off-loads ionized calcium increasing the amount of biologically active calcium in the serum in the presence of acidosis. This is the rationale behind rebreathing to increase CO_2 retention and a respiratory acidosis to help compensate for the acute deficiency in ionized serum calcium. Cardiac abnormalities are also present in hypercalcemia, such as that seen in the rare situation referred to as "parathyroid poisoning". In this instance, however, with excess calcium there is failure to relax following muscle contraction. This is reflected in the unusual cardiac manifestation of systolic arrest, which is a terminal event of hypercalcemic crisis.

Items 17-20

    (A)   General anesthesia
    (B)   Regional anesthesia
    (C)   Both
    (D)   Neither

17. can cause hypotension

18. muscle relaxation

19. requires intravenous access

20. patient can often hear and remember

Items 21-24

    (A)   Hypoxemia
    (B)   Hypercarbia
    (C)   Both
    (D)   Neither

21. agitation

22. anesthesia at significant levels

23. respiratory drive

24. dangerous in neurosurgery

ANSWERS AND TUTORIAL ON ITEMS 17-20

The answers are: **17-C; 18-A; 19-C; 20-C**.

    The choice of regional versus general anesthesia is sometimes made on the assumption that regional anesthesia is somehow less invasive and disturbs the patient's physiology less, so that the patient can be left alone as far as ventilation and circulation are concerned when only "one leg is put to sleep." Apart from the consequences of a high spinal and its respiratory consequences, spinal anesthesia causes a major change in circulation, with paralysis of the capacitance reservoirs allowing peripheral pooling of blood. General anesthesia can also cause peripheral pooling by vasodilatation, so both may lead to hypotension without careful fluid support of circulation. Neither should be attempted without intravenous access.

It is also thought that with regional anesthesia such as axillary block, intravenous lidocaine with tourniquet, spinal or epidural anesthesia, a patient can hear and remember events in the operation even if some supplementary neuroleptic agent is given. This is true. But it is also true for general anesthesia in which the patient may have lost consciousness at induction but certainly has lost ability to express what he hears or feels when paralyzed and intubated. It is often the case that patients can relate vividly details of the events that have occurred, particularly toward arousal from anesthesia, and often express less fear than alarm and offense at apparently callous behavior and remarks. Protection of the operative team is not an indication for the choice of anesthetic! In this instance, behavior modification would be more appropriate to continually consider each patient as you would yourself, monitoring the activity of each.

ANSWERS AND TUTORIAL ON ITEMS 21-24

The answers are: **21-A; 22-C; 23-C; 24-C**.

The patient who is agitated and difficult to quiet must never be assured, sedated or dismissed until hypoxemia is ruled out! One does not sleep or "rest comfortably" when one's adrenals are squeezed in a survival response, and hypoxemia is a serious fixable etiology for restlessness and complaints disturbing the nursing staff. If the clinician should give orders for sedation to the patient who is combative, pulling tubes and smashing bottles, hypoxemia can be converted to anoxia with lethal consequence. Hypoxemia must first be ruled out before any management method that might not resolve it or make it worse.

Hypercarbia has the opposite effect, and at higher levels of CO_2 tension, carbon dioxide is anesthetic. The combination of hypercarbia and hypoxia is a highly effective anesthetic with no margin of safety between anesthesia and death. This maxim has been proven with a practice to be discouraged in which dental procedures or other short operations were performed following ninety seconds of pure nitrous oxide ventilation. This was intended to produce what was euphemistically called "nitrous cyanosis" which meant that the effective anesthesia under which the tooth was pulled was hypercarbic anoxia. No one should require closer experience with death in a dental chair than by this observation to take necessary preventive precautions.

Both hypoxemia and hypercarbia are respiratory drives. Over time, the patient who loses sensitivity to hypercarbia through CO_2 retention in chronic lung disease survives almost exclusively on the hypoxic drive which is why a short course of inhalation oxygen can stop such a patient breathing when the anesthetic role of hypercarbia takes over.

Hypercarbia is dangerous in patients with head injury, since cerebral blood flow is sensitive to CO_2 tension. Hyperventilation of the patient with a closed head injury can prevent rapid and progressive cerebral edema, and a continuous maintenance of appropriate oxygen tensions is the only way to maintain vitality in the brain — since there are no oxygen stores, no readily available alternate metabolic pathways other than aerobic metabolism, and no energy stores for glycolysis in this vital organ dependant on minute to minute delivery of oxygen.

Items 25-28

    (A) Ketoacidosis
    (B) Insulin shock
    (C) Both
    (D) Neither

25. 50 ml 50% glucose push IV is harmful

26. coma

27. potassium therapy

28. Kussmaul respirations

Items 29-33

    (A) Melanoma
    (B) Dermatofibroma
    (C) Erysipelas
    (D) Neurofibroma
    (E) Rodent ulcer
    (F) Junctional nevus
    (G) Actinic keratosis

29. *Streptococcus* is an etiologic factor.

30. May occur in families with other features of a recognized syndrome.

31. A pigmented mole with premalignant potential.

32. Squamous cell cancer is a consequence.

33. Characteristically spreads to lymph nodes.

ANSWERS AND TUTORIAL ON ITEMS 25-28

The answers are: **25-D; 26-C; 27-C; 28-A**.

In a diabetic patient who presents in coma, either too little or too much insulin may have resulted in too much or too little blood sugar. Kussmaul respiration is indicative of diabetic coma and the aroma of ketones being hyperventilated may be helpful. However, a blood sugar determination may be drawn, but results not awaited before a simple differentiation by a therapeutic test.

It would be very dangerous to inject insulin to see if that would help differentiate the two sources of coma in the diabetic, and the results would be neither immediate nor definitive. However, this is not the case with the obverse. An IV push of 50 ml of 50% glucose abruptly awakens the patient in the event of hypoglycemic coma and will not significantly harm the patient if this diagnostic test turns out not to be correct. This is one of the simplest, most dramatic and commonest of the instances in which the therapy for disease precedes diagnosis or is its equivalent.

Potassium therapy should accompany treatment for either condition, since administration of insulin will drive both sugar and potassium into the cell and might result in dangerous hypokalemia. The two extremes of coma in the diabetic can be safely differentiated by a trial pulse of glucose which will dramatically help in one instance confirming the diagnosis and will not harm the patient if the coma is due to the alternate problem of too little insulin effect.

ANSWERS AND TUTORIAL ON ITEMS 29-33

The answers are: **29-C; 30-D; 31-F; 32-G; 33-A**.

Erysipelas is a superficial cellulitis that spreads with the rapidity of streptococcal infections and the associated enzymes that prevent the body from walling off and containing them. It is a lesion that is inflammatory and infectious, and distinct from the other acquired lumps or moles in this list in that it has a clinically recognizable pattern that is treatable by antibiotic and local therapy. Two of these skin lumps have fibroma as a component of their names, but the one is of neurofibroma origin and may occur in a familial syndrome with other abnormalities known as von Recklinghausen syndrome.

There are some lesions here that are malignant and some that are premalignant, and actinic keratosis is one that is cutaneous in exposed areas of the body in which sunlight or X-irradiation has been a chronic stimulus, and squamous cell carcinoma is the malignant consequence of actinic keratosis. There are two pigmented mole lesions, the one being junctional nevus, and it has a premalignant potential in the junctional component of the mole. When it becomes malignant, it degenerates to melanoma (a threat distinctly absent in the other pigmented mole with which it can be confused, compound nevus) and the characteristic dissemination of melanoma is through lymphatic metastases.

Items 34-38

    (A) Hypovolemic shock
    (B) Cardiogenic shock
    (C) Peripheral pooling
    (D) Endotoxic shock

34. high fluid volume and transfusion harmful

35. seen after spinal anesthesia

36. cellular defect in metabolism

37. pericardial tamponade

38. warm pink extremities with bounding pulse

Items 39-43

Hemostasis by:

    (A) Lavage
    (B) Arteriographic pressor or embolus
    (C) Tamponade (e.g., packing, balloon)
    (D) Sclerotherapy
    (E) Diathermy
    (F) Laser
    (G) Actual (hot) cautery
    (H) Topical pharmacology (e.g., collagen constrictors)
    (I) Ligation
    (J) Expectant therapy

39. control of accessible artery by operative exposure

40. retinal hemorrhage

41. recommended for split thickness skin graft donor site

42. injection technique via endoscopy

43. management method for crush fracture pelvis

ANSWERS AND TUTORIAL ON ITEMS 34-38

The answers are: **34-B; 35-C; 36-D; 37-B; 38-D**.

Shock is a state of insufficient nutrient flow, and adequate nutrient flow is necessary for aerobic metabolism. The markers of insufficiency or non-nutrient flow include the products of anaerobic metabolism and incomplete glucose breakdown — hydrogen ion, lactate and pyruvate. Each of these conditions, to be called "shock", share the common feature of insufficient nutrient flow, and all are marked by the anaerobic metabolic features.

Hypovolemic shock may be among the most common (and was the first type recognized and treated), but it is not the only form of shock, and if all shock is treated as hypovolemia, volume therapy is actually harmful to cardiogenic shock in which the volume is not insufficient but the capability of delivering that volume is. Another form of cardiogenic shock is the interference in venous return that may occur with pericardial tamponade, making the insufficiency not so much a form of inadequate cardiac contraction but of inadequate ventricular volume to be propelled.

Spinal anesthesia may paralyze the capacitance venous reservoirs that dilate and make for an effective subtraction in the circulating volume. A similar phenomenon occurs with neurogenic shock, sequestering volume that would otherwise be in circulation. Endotoxic shock is a form of cellular defect in which the cells are not using the nutrients delivered to them because of a cytochrome inactivation such as some poisons (cyanide, endotoxin) or an inability to get either glucose or oxygen inside the cell (diabetes, carbon monoxide poisoning). This is a form of shock for which recognition is counterintuitive, since the extremities may be warm and pink with the nailbeds apparently well perfused and bounding pulses palpable in the extremities. Despite the high cardiac output from the low peripheral vascular resistance, the cells are in shock and reflect this with an accumulating hydrogen ion burden that generally causes this high cardiac output to decrease when acidosis neutralizes the catecholamine compensation.

ANSWERS AND TUTORIAL ON ITEMS 39-43

The answers are: **39-I; 40-F; 41-C; 42-D; 43-B**.

The method of control of bleeding is determined by the type of vessel bleeding and the exposure to it for application of energy via various techniques. For example, a retinal hemorrhage has really only recently had pinpoint precision control through laser photocoagulation. For a bleeding artery that is accessible by means of surgical exposure, ligature remains the most secure and reliable method of hemostasis. If the bleeding site can be seen and the pressure propelling the hemorrhage is less than full systolic arterial pressure, sclerotherapy may be successful in such positions as the esophagus or lower GI tract via endoscopic technique. Direct pressure application is often sufficient for end vessel bleeding as occurs with the donor site of a split thickness skin graft. Although various dressings have been promoted that have some pharmacologic agent or collagen or other clot promoter impregnated in them, the active ingredient is the application of topical pressure for hemostasis.

A very vexing problem of multiple trauma is the hemorrhage that is experienced with pelvic fractures from crush injury. One of the more successful techniques to date for this combined venous and arterial bleeding from the efferent side that cannot be exposed or controlled is the use of arteriographic therapy, infusing constrictors or occasionally even embolizing the feeding arterial vessel to decrease the perfusion pressure associated with the fracture site bleeding.

Items 44-48

(A) Arterial pressure
(B) Venous pressure
(C) Lymphatic pressure
(D) Gut luminal pressure

44. primarily responsible for perforation

45. first mural vessel to have elevated pressure in bowel obstruction

46. increasing pressure does *not* lead to stasis

47. blue congestion macroscopically, diapedesis microscopically

48. primarily responsible for edema

ANSWERS AND TUTORIAL ON ITEMS 44-48

The answers are: **44-D; 45-C; 46-A; 47-B; 48-C**.

In mechanical or functional bowel obstruction, the intraluminal pressure in the gut rises from both secretions entering it and the propulsion of those secretions along its length. It is the luminal pressure that first rises and is ultimately responsible for perforation of the gastrointestinal tract, usually at a point weakened by necrosis after all other vascular pressures within the bowel wall have been elevated to the intraluminal pressure. The first of these mural vessels to experience increased pressure is the lymphatic system. It is the lymphatic pressure increase that is primarily responsible for edema, with transudation of plasma evident in a boggy pale and thickened bowel. The next pressure elevation in the next lowest system of intraluminal vessel pressures is the vein, and when venous hypertension sets in translated through from the greater resistance imparted by the edematous bowel from lymphatic pressure rise, blood cells now pass through the vessel walls as well as the plasma "weeping" that had started earlier with the lymphatic and early venous pressure rise. This makes the bowel blue and congested in appearance macroscopically. In microscopic appearance, the passage of red cells through the wall is recognized as diapedesis. Stasis occurs stopping all blood flow when venous pressure rises to arterial pressure, and since the arterial perfusion is the highest pressure system, a further rise in its pressure is the only rise that would not contribute to stasis of perfusion.

Items 49-53

Deficiencies in:

    (A)   Factor VIII
    (B)   Factor IX
    (C)   Factor XIII
    (D)   Calcium
    (E)   Silk ligature

49. deficiency that is the most frequent cause of postoperative hemorrhage

50. chelation is anticoagulant

51. Christmas disease

52. von Willebrand's disease

53. classic hemophilia

ANSWERS AND TUTORIAL ON ITEMS 49-53

The answers are: **49-E; 50-D; 51-B; 52-C; 53-A.**

    Calcium is a necessary factor in the clotting cascade, and it is by chelating calcium that most donated blood is able to be stored in refrigerated bags without clotting. The anticoagulant in most donated blood, therefore, carries this ability to continue binding calcium, and multiple unit transfusions should consider the possibility that calcium deficiency would result after the equivalent of the fifth unit of banked blood with its citrate anticoagulant binding calcium. Factor VIII deficiency causes classic hemophilia, and infusions of this factor can prevent the spontaneous hemorrhage with minimal trauma such as that seen in joints of the hemophiliac patient.

Factor IX deficiency gives an atypical hemophilia referred to as Christmas disease named after the family in which it was first isolated, and Factor IX therapy is corrective for this deficiency. Factor XIII deficiency is referred to as von Willebrand's disease, and has more to do with vascular fragility than with a missing protocoagulant.

Of all the sources of bleeding encountered postoperatively, the deficiency most commonly responsible for the bleeding is "acute silk deficiency" — that is, failure to achieve effective ligation of bleeding vessels.

Items 54-58

(A) Insufficient clotting
(B) Ineffective clotting
(C) Excess clotting
(D) Excessive fibrinolysis
(E) Platelet abnormalities
(F) Circulating anticoagulants

54. therapy with aminocaproic acid

55. disseminated intravascular coagulation

56. amniotic fluid embolus hypofibrinogenemia

57. prolonged partial thromboplastin tissue

58. prolonged prothrombin time

ANSWERS AND TUTORIAL ON ITEMS 54-58

The answers are: **54-D; 55-C; 56-A; 57-F; 58-A**.

The list of options includes most sources of uncontrolled postoperative bleeding. If there are inadequate prothrombin factors (such as by consumption of these labile factors or because of deficiency in their production because of hepatic insufficiency or coumadin poisoning of their production), clotting will be insufficient. That is also true if there is inadequate fibrinogen, and that may occur from such sources as rapid consumption in the event of infusion of amniotic fluid in peripartum amniotic embolus.) In each of these events and in one more generalized one called disseminated intravascular coagulation, the reserve supply of labile clotting factors is consumed, and bleeding thereafter is uncontrolled by effective clotting in a quantity sufficient to maintain control after securing bleeding vessels.

In order to allow restoration of these clotting factors to the level where they can sustain effective clotting in sufficient quantity, some bleeding patients are paradoxically treated with anticoagulation to reduce the consumption until an additional means of local control is added and the anticoagulation stopped or reversed so that the clotting cascade can resume. ← heparin

The other sources of excessive bleeding include circulating anticoagulant, and that would give rise to a partial thromboplastin time that was prolonged as evidence that it might be one origin of the bleeding problem. An additional factor might be the premature dissolution of clots by excessive plasminogen activator activity. To slow down clot dissolution by plasminogen activator, aminocaproic acid can be used therapeutically to prolong the life of fibrin clot. It is important to state again that each of these maneuvers are considered after local surgical control has been achieved or has failed after a thorough attempt because of some systemic problem, but focal bleeding from an open vessel is not treated by factor therapy.

heparin induced PTT

Items 59-63

- (A) Oral erythromycin base and neomycin
- (B) Oral penicillin
- (C) Oral chloramphenicol
- (D) Intravenous cefoxitin
- (E) Intravenous cefazolin
- (F) Intravenous imipenem
- (G) Topical sulfamylon
- (H) Topical iodophores (Betadine)
- (I) Irrigation with dilute (Dakan's) hypochlorite
- (J) None of the above

59. associated with aplastic anemia

60. induces brisk catharsis

61. appropriate systemic prophylaxis for elective colon resection

62. appropriate prophylaxis initiated in the postoperative recovery room

63. preferred treatment following full thickness burn escharectomy

ANSWERS AND TUTORIAL ON ITEMS 59-63

The answers are: **59-C; 60-A; 61-D; 62-J; 63-G.**

Oral erythromycin base and neomycin are considered "pipe cleaners", i.e., minimally absorbable antibiotics, that largely exert their affect in the colon where floral populations are highest. One of the effective means of colon preparation stemming from the use of these antibiotics is that they induce a brisk mechanical bowel purging from their cathartic effect. Another oral antibiotic that would be effective against the principle flora of the colon (the predominant *Bacteroides* and other anaerobic gram-negative species) would be oral chloramphenicol. However, this antibiotic is absorbable, and has been associated with the catastrophe of aplastic anemia that is rare but lethal. The same antibiotic injected by vein does not seem to give rise to this complication as often, therefore the utility of chloramphenicol in the hospitalized patient should be limited to non-oral use.

Topical therapy can be employed for reducing inoculum in large denuded surfaces, such as that which occurs in burn patients following excision of devitalized tissue and eschar. Sulfamylon is appropriate therapy for such denudation since it has good local flora control on surface contamination with less significant effects of absorption than other topical agents that have also been employed.

Prophylaxis is mandated in procedures in which the inoculum cannot be adequately prevented or there is high risk such as prosthetic implantation in patients undergoing elective operation. Surface and intracavitary decontamination is attempted, but in the colon the flora are so numerous that intravenous antibiotic prophylaxis is appropriate, particularly selecting an agent that would be active against the flora most likely to be encountered. Intravenous cefoxitin fulfills these requirements, and is appropriate as prophylaxis for elective colon resection.

Although intravenous imipenem might have a broad spectrum and high effectiveness, it should never be used in prophylaxis to guard its utility as a highly effective antibiotic monotherapy in seriously ill patients. If widely used in such instances as prophylaxis, when patient benefit is marginal, its effectiveness as an antibiotic might be compromised by generating bacterial resistance.

By definition, prophylaxis is that antibiotic that is circulating before the inoculum, and therefore, there is no prophylaxis claim that can justify the use of an antibiotic first employed postoperatively. To be employed following operation, an antibiotic must be justified on a therapeutic claim, and this would require clinical evidence, (fever chart, urinalysis, chest X ray, white blood count elevation) or microbiologic evidence (Gram stain, culture and sensitivity). Prophylaxis is prospective, and there is a contradiction in terms in the use of prophylaxis in the context of trauma or postoperative events. Unless the antimicrobial employed is circulating before the inoculum that cannot be prevented, its use fails the definition of prophylaxis.

Items 64-68

- (A) Whole blood
- (B) Packed red cells
- (C) Fresh frozen single donor plasma
- (D) Human serum albumin
- (E) Plasmanate
- (F) D_5/Ringer's lactate
- (G) D_5/W
- (H) Normal saline
- (I) Platelet pack concentrate

64. treatment of anemia

65. rapid sequestration in hypersplenism

66. inappropriate resuscitation fluid for recent trauma victim

67. most frequently used infusion for trauma

68. can produce seizures in head injured patient

ANSWERS AND TUTORIAL ON ITEMS 64-68

The answers are: **64-B; 65-I; 66-C; 67-F; 68-G.**

Each of these infusion or transfusion fluids is used in resuscitation selected on the basis of the predominant utility of crystalloid, colloid, or red cell mass. The treatment of anemia requires hemoglobin, and the most efficient way that is distributed is in red cells. Whole blood should be used extremely rarely, since it has more functional utility when divided into components and the component is selected for a patient deficit in that function. Of the several colloids, fresh frozen single donor plasma may have abundant labile coagulating factors contained within it, but should not be used as resuscitation for a recent trauma victim who has no demonstrated deficit in any of these factors as yet.

The most frequently used fluid for trauma victims is crystalloid solution such as Ringer's Lactate. One of the types of trauma that may be encountered is closed head trauma which may exhibit the unusual affect of retaining water excessively and dilutional hyponatremia. This is especially true in the unusual syndrome that may follow some forms of intracranial injury called "the syndrome of inappropriate diuretic hormone" (SIADH). Moreover, an excess water volume will lead to cerebral edema, and free water clearance ought to be encouraged in these patients, most generally by fluid restriction.

Platelet pack concentrate is a highly specialized infusion of fresh platelets from several donors after separation from the plasma which can be employed for multiple other factor extractions and then pooled colloid content. In a patient who has platelet deficit, this may help raise platelets to adequate clotting level, but will not relieve the patient of the source of thrombocytopenia to begin with. In the event that the patient continues to have hypersplenism as platelets are administered, those platelets will be rapidly sequestered in the spleen and will drop off rapidly unless a platelet transfusion is a component part of surgical therapy or at least medical suppression of the hypersplenic activity.

Items 69-73

(A) Gram-positive aerobes
(B) Gram-negative aerobes
(C) Gram-negative anaerobes
(D) Protozoa
(E) Viruses

69. cellulitis and superficial abscess

70. endotoxemia

71. late intra-abdominal abscess

72. pneumonia in HIV positive patients

73. commonest skin flora

ANSWERS AND TUTORIAL ON ITEMS 69-73

The answers are: **69-A; 70-B; 71-C; 72-D; 73-A**.

Gram-positive aerobic agents (*Staphylococci* and *Streptococci*) are among the commonest of the skin flora, and are responsible for cellulitis and superficial abscess formation in any break in the first line of defense and exposure of the interior milieu to these skin flora. In contrast, gram-negative aerobes are the flora associated with endotoxin release and the high mortality of endotoxemia in contrast with the morbidity of skin flora in causing cellulitis and abscess.

Late in the mixed inoculum, intra-abdominal abscess is predominately a factor of anaerobic proliferation, since the more numerous anaerobes gradually outgrow the aerobes. The mixed aerobic and anaerobic flora are synergistic, since micro-aerophilic circumstances later in an abscess favor a higher number of anaerobes that survive from the original mixed inoculum.

One protozoan organism, *Pneumocystis carinii* has a predilection for patients with immunocompromise, which includes those with HIV infection. The HIV is not responsible for the pneumonia, but for the immunosuppressed status that allows the protozoan pneumonia to become established.

Items 74-78

(A) *Staphylococcus aureus*
(B) β-hemolytic *Streptococcus*
(C) *Hemophilus influenza*
(D) *Escherichia coli*
(E) *Proteus mirabilis*
(F) *Pseudomonas aeruginosa*
(G) *Clostridium perfringens*
(H) *Clostridium difficile*
(I) *Bacteroides fragilis*

74. Earliest widespread infecting organism of spreading cellulitis.

75. Associated with pseudomembranous colitis.

76. Organism frequently found in humidifiers of ventilators.

77. Most numerous species by weight in colon contents.

78. Most common organism cultured from urinary tract infections.

ANSWERS AND TUTORIAL ON ITEMS 74-78

The answers are: **74-B; 75-H; 76-F; 77-I; 78-D**.

Cellulitis due to β-hemolytic streptococci spreads because of the enzymatic activity of this organism, and the inability of the host to wall it off as frequently occurs with staphylococcal infections that can be limited to abscesses. Of the gram-negative anaerobes, *Bacteroides* are the most numerous, constituting the majority of the dry weight of colon contents. Clostridia are also present in this class of gram-negative anaerobes, and *Clostridium difficile* secretes an exotoxin which is associated with pseudomembranous colitis. One of the organisms found in the damp environments of ventilators, particularly in the humidifiers, is *Pseudomonas aeruginosa*. It is particularly hard to eradicate without sterilizing this equipment by complete disassembly between patients.

The urinary tract is not an anaerobic environment. In essence, one does not need to concern oneself about the likelihood of upper urinary tract infection with any species other than the gram-negative aerobe. The lower urinary tract has the likelihood of skin flora invasion, which is what happens frequently with indwelling catheters, as a channel between the flora of the skin conducted into the mucosal environment of peri-urethritis.

That the mixed flora of the gut is mainly anaerobic and the pathogens responsible for urinary tract infections are principally coliforms means that therapy can be tailored to avoid impact on the most numerous species of the gut so as to minimize GI flora disturbance in such anaerobe sparing therapy as quinolone treatment. For example, norfloxacin might be given with minimal gastrointestinal flora upset and cover the majority of risks to urinary tract colonizing organisms.

Items 79-83

- (A) Morphine
- (B) Nitrous oxide
- (C) Epidural tetracaine
- (D) Spinal anesthetic
- (E) Local infiltration lidocaine/epinephrine
- (F) Axillary block regional
- (G) Alcohol nerve block
- (H) Sympathectomy

79. may be useful for plastic surgery procedure in hemostasis

80. may temporarily increase marginal blood flow to a limb threatened by small vessel disease

81. reversed by naloxone

82. may be useful for 72 hours postoperative analgesia with minimum respiratory depression

83. may be helpful in long-term control of chronic cancer pain

ANSWERS AND TUTORIAL ON ITEMS 79-83

The answers are: **79-E; 80-H; 81-A; 82-C; 83-G**.

Anesthesia and analgesia are tailored to the indication, duration, and procedure. In some plastic surgical procedures, anesthesia by infiltration injection by the surgeon performing the procedure is actually preferred, since the injection of lidocaine may give local anesthesia, but the combination with epinephrine may actually reduce skin bleeding and facilitate primary closure. It is important that this use of vasoconstriction be employed only in tissues that would not be impaired by it to the degree that they might suffer ischemia and infarction if they are supplied by end vessels; this would include those on tip of the nose, and cartilaginous portions of the ear or flaps with marginal and compromised blood flow.

Regional nerve block may be done by a temporary method using reversible pharmacology, or may actually attempt destruction of the nerve for a longer term relief of pain. Injection of alcohol in sensory nerve block after demonstration of its effect using short-term anesthetic agents may be useful in long-term control of intractable cancer pain. Similarly, by either surgical sympathectomy or pharmacologic ablation using similar techniques as that for cancer pain control in sensory nerves, sympathectomy may allow — at least for a period of months — an increased blood flow to a marginally supplied extremity in threatened limb loss.

Morphine, with its excellent analgesic properties, carries with it some risk of respiratory depression as well as associated nausea and some properties such as histamine release or stimulation of sphincter spasm at pancreatic or biliary outlet. For that reason, on some occasions, morphine analgesia may not be just inappropriate, but there may be therapeutic benefit to reversing it with naloxone as an opioid antagonist. In order to achieve analgesia over a prolonged period of time without the respiratory hazard particularly observed with the use of morphine and its associated obtundation, an epidural catheter can be placed and infused with a dilute analgesic for a period of time indwelling in the epidural space. Since the catheter might constitute a channel for skin flora to contaminate this space in which an abscess would be very hazardous, it is not suggested that such an indwelling epidural catheter remain over a very extensive period, but usually this is satisfactory for the period of most intense postoperative pain when respiratory suppression would be most hazardous, and the catheter can be pulled and this form of analgesic substituted for by systemic analgesia when the patient is ambulating and at less risk for various consequences of respiratory suppression.

Items 84-93

84. Mechanical bowel preparation can be accomplished through all of the following means **EXCEPT**:

    (A) oral administration of an osmotic solution
    (B) instillation of saline solution through a nasogastric tube
    (C) oral neomycin and erythromycin-base antibiotic administration
    (D) intramuscular broad-spectrum cephalosporin administration
    (E) oil retention enema

85. Surface decontamination in pre-operative preparation of the surgical field has demonstrated which of the following methods of hair removal is microbiologically superior with a lower risk of surgical wound infection?

    (A) no hair removal
    (B) electric clipper
    (C) dry shaving with razor
    (D) lather scrub and razor shave
    (E) depilatory cream

86. Which of the following statements is true regarding a comparison of antibiotic monotherapy using imipenem in comparison with combination therapy with clindamycin and tobramycin in septic surgical patients?

    (A) imipenem monotherapy is superior to combination therapy in all septic patients studied
    (B) combination therapy is superior to imipenem monotherapy in all patients studied
    (C) combination therapy is superior to imipenem monotherapy in only the sickest group of patients under study
    (D) imipenem monotherapy is superior to combination therapy only in the sickest patients under study
    (E) combination antibiotic therapy is the equivalent of imipenem monotherapy in all patients studied

87. Antibiotic prophylaxis is **NOT** indicated in which of the following patient settings?

    (A) elective colon resection for carcinoma
    (B) implantation of hip prosthesis
    (C) aortic valve replacement
    (D) thyroidectomy for invasive thyroid cancer
    (E) hemorrhoidectomy in patient with rheumatic heart disease

88. The most frequent organisms in highest density that can be isolated from contamination following colon perforation are

 (A) gram-positive aerobes
 (B) gram-negative aerobes
 (C) gram-positive anaerobes
 (D) gram-negative anaerobes
 (E) protozoan organisms

89. Which of the following groups of microflora are associated with endotoxemia?

 (A) gram-positive aerobes
 (B) gram-negative aerobes
 (C) gram-positive anaerobes
 (D) gram-negative anaerobes
 (E) protozoan organisms

90. Pseudomembranous colitis is associated with which group of microorganisms?

 (A) *Staphylococcus*
 (B) *Streptococcus*
 (C) coliforms
 (D) *Pseudomonas*
 (E) *Clostridium*

91. The preferred treatment of an infected foreign body implanted in musculoskeletal tissue is

 (A) removal of the foreign body
 (B) antibiotic therapy with gram-positive aerobic coverage
 (C) implantation of impregnated beads that release antibiotic effective against gram-negative aerobes
 (D) irrigation through adjacent catheters with oxidizing solutions
 (E) unroofing and exposure of the infected site for granulation

92. Monoclonal anti-endotoxin therapy has been used in patients with results best characterized by which of the following?

 (A) only patients with positive blood cultures benefitted
 (B) only patients with higher severity of illness scores benefitted
 (C) patients were benefitted only if the agents were administered before shock set in
 (D) no benefit was seen if the patient had a negative assay for endotoxemia
 (E) patient benefits could not be discriminated based on measurable parameters of sepsis or their mediators

93. An organism frequently cultured from indwelling hyperalimentation subclavian catheters in immunosuppressed patients on broad spectrum antibiotics is

   (A)   *Pneumocystis carinii*
   (B)   *Mycobacterium tuberculosis*
   (C)   *Bacteroides fragilis*
   (D)   *Pseudomonas aeruginosa*
   (E)   *Candida albicans*

ANSWERS AND TUTORIALS ON ITEMS 84-93

The answers are: **84-D; 85-A; 86-D; 87-D; 88-D; 89-B; 90-E; 91-A; 92-E; 93-E**.

84. Bowel preparation involves the "pipe cleaners" of nonabsorbable antibiotics which cause brisk catharsis, as does oral administration of osmotic solutions or a saline load or enema use. Systemic administration of cephalosporins may give antibiotic effect where the circulation carries them, but that does not include the resident flora within the gut.

85. If an experimental model were designed to enhance the probability of wound infection, it would be hard to surpass the "standard of care" written into nursing procedure manuals for operating room routines. First, a patient impaired by a disease process and often nutritionally deficient is administered immunosuppressive drugs, then the stratum corneum is scraped off with a razor, denuding the first line of defense. With the excoriations and superficial burns lowering cutaneous resistance, this injured barrier is then recolonized with hospital flora — a group of pathogens selected for its resistance to most commonly used treatment regimens.

With this microflora now established in the injured barrier, further insult comes from scrubbing the burn with a brush, mechanical shearing forces and toxic chemical solutions. An incision is then made through this previously intact resistant barrier to infection.

The best microbiologic protection comes from no hair removal at all at operative incisions. This is particularly critical at such sites as eyebrows, which, once shaved, do not often grow back. If hair must be removed for exposure for the incision or for adherent draping or dressing, the method that least injures skin should be favored — clipping being the next best — which nonetheless leaves a supracuticular stubble.

86. In the most inclusive and carefully controlled antibiotic trial ever conducted for collaborative evaluation of surgical sepsis regimens, imipenem monotherapy was shown to be the equivalent of combination aminoglycoside (tobramycin, in this study) and anti-anaerobic drug (clindamycin in this study) for patients at lesser severity of illness ratings. But, for patients who were significantly more ill, particularly with multiple organ failure onset, monotherapy was significantly superior to combination therapy.

The important feature of this study that set a standard for future clinical trials of antibiotic regimens in surgical sepsis, is that patients must be stratified according to severity of illness for any meaningful outcome results in comparing treatments.

87. Clean elective surgical procedures do not require antibiotic prophylaxis unless there is a high inoculum that cannot be removed by preparation (as is often the case in colon resections), or there is prosthetic material with a local site of reduced resistance (as is true for orthopedic or cardiac prostheses), or there is impaired resistance from an area with natural immunity defect (such as rheumatic valve disease). Thyroid cancer does not constitute a considerable immunologic deficiency, and the inoculum should be negligible following skin preparation in the elective thyroidectomy.

88. Gram-negative anaerobes are the most numerous species in the lower GI tract and can make up to 80% of the dry weight of fecal contents. Other flora are present in the mixed inoculum but with much lower frequency.

89. Endotoxins are products of the coliform class of microorganisms of which *E. coli* is the prototype. Some of the gram-positive organisms and a few of the gram-negative anaerobes may be associated with exotoxins, but endotoxemia is a characteristic associated with gram-negative aerobic sepsis.

90. *Clostridium* is a gram-negative anaerobe, and one species, *Clostridium difficile*, is associated with the production of an exotoxin responsible for the development of pseudomembranous colitis.

91. The treatment of an infected foreign body is its removal. If the foreign body is a prosthesis that is necessary for function, that function must be either bypassed extraanatomically or replaced after eradication of the infection. Antibiotic therapy alone will not clear the source of sepsis if the foreign body remains.

92. Monoclonal antibody therapy had potential promise in patients suffering endotoxemic shock; however, clinical trials of these agents could not discriminate benefit based on positive or negative blood cultures, endotoxin assays, or severity of illness, and without these indications for rational administration, this class of agents has not yet been approved by the FDA for general use.

93. Immunosuppressed patients may be susceptible to *Pneumocystis* or tuberculosis, but they do not get it typically as catheter sepsis. Although both *Bacteroides* and *Pseudomonas* are possible, they would not be likely in the setting described. *Candida albicans* is the fungus which is most likely in the setting of the immunosuppressed patient given prolonged antibiotics and hyperosmotic total parenteral nutrition fluid and is a recognized source of catheter sepsis.

Items 94-103

94. In setting oxygen tension, ventilatory rate, and tidal volume for ventilator therapy, the best clinical setting would be one that achieves

    (A) a tidal volume of 700 ml
    (B) a positive end expiratory pressure of 25 cm of water
    (C) an arterial partial pressure of oxygen of 450 mm Hg
    (D) a pH of 7.62
    (E) arterial oxygen saturation of 90%

95. A negative and undesirable effect of positive end expiratory pressure (PEEP) would be

    (A) decrease physiologic shunting
    (B) improve compliance
    (C) decrease venous return
    (D) improve arterial partial pressure of oxygen
    (E) decrease inspired oxygen

96. Candidates for transient extrapulmonary assistance in oxygenation are those patients with severe but reversible pulmonary insufficiency which would include

    (A) *Pneumocystis carinii* pneumonia
    (B) bronchiectasis
    (C) emphysema
    (D) pulmonary fibrosis
    (E) pneumoconiosis

97. Oxygen inhalation therapy by nasal prongs is contraindicated in which of the following conditions?

    (A) chronic emphysema
    (B) acute pulmonary edema
    (C) diplococcal pneumonia
    (D) myocardial infarction
    (E) *Pneumocystis carinii* pneumonia

98. A Stage I epidermoid lung carcinoma in the right upper lobe of a patient with chronic emphysema and a 60 mm Hg oxygen tension on 40% assisted oxygen ventilation in a patient dependant on the ventilator represents a situation in which there is a/an

    (A) resectable tumor in an operable patient
    (B) nonresectable tumor in an operable patient
    (C) resectable tumor in an inoperable patient
    (D) nonresectable tumor in an inoperable patient
    (E) indication for expeditious thoracotomy and lobectomy

99. Pulmonary emphysema occurring at an early age of onset is associated with

    (A) mucoviscidosis
    (B) congenital atresia of the opposite lung
    (C) alpha-1 antitrypsin deficiency
    (D) acetylcysteine therapy
    (E) tracheoesophageal fistula

100. Pneumonia secondary to aspiration of gastric contents is a complication frequently seen in all of the following patient conditions **EXCEPT**:

    (A) laryngectomy
    (B) chronic alcoholism
    (C) closed head injury
    (D) heroin addiction
    (E) infant asthma

101. Thromboembolism is **LEAST** likely in which clinical setting?

    (A) hip fracture
    (B) paraplegia
    (C) prolonged abdominal pelvic operation
    (D) polycythemia
    (E) thrombocytopenia

102. Bronchospasm is treated by each of the following maneuvers **EXCEPT**:

    (A) rigorous endotracheal suctioning
    (B) β-adrenergic drugs
    (C) somatostatin analog
    (D) short-acting muscle paralysis
    (E) long-acting muscle relaxation

103. Tube thoracostomy is employed in each of the following procedures **EXCEPT**:

　　(A)　total right pneumonectomy
　　(B)　spontaneous pneumothorax
　　(C)　chylothorax
　　(D)　right upper lobectomy
　　(E)　hemothorax from multiple rib fractures

ANSWERS AND TUTORIALS ON ITEMS 94-103

The answers are: **94-E; 95-C; 96-A; 97-A; 98-C; 99-C; 100-A; 101-E; 102-A; 103-A**.

94. Hemoglobin is the most efficient oxygen carrier known, and once 90% saturation is achieved, the greater oxygen tensions result in very little additional oxygen carriage at much higher toxicity. Alkalosis inhibits oxygen release from oxyhemoglobin. Tidal volume depends on patient size and dead space that is subtracted from it, and end expiratory pressures would be appropriate depending on the positive benefit in reduction of physiologic shunt with minimal impact on venous return and cardiac output. Oxygen saturation of hemoglobin would be the appropriate indicator of clinical ventilator support.

95. PEEP improves the oxygen tension in any given quantity of blood flowing through the pulmonary veins by decreasing pulmonary shunting and improving compliance. However, the positive pressure that affects a greater amount of air in the lungs also affects the low pressure systemic venous blood return and thereby may reduce cardiac output. A greater concentration of oxygen is therefore carried, but in a lesser output of arterialized blood. Early stages of PEEP maximize the beneficial effects, but much higher levels impair delivery of this improved oxygen concentration in a smaller output from the heart.

96. *Pneumocystis carinii* pneumonia is an acute pneumonitis with severe respiratory insufficiency and inability to oxygenate blood with the affected lungs; however, there is an antimicrobial therapy which is effective over a short period of time, and no structural damage is residual in the lung, so such patients could be weaned from extracorporeal oxygenation and back to pulmonary respiration. Pulmonary fibrosis, pneumoconiosis, bronchiectasis and emphysema are all architectural changes with nonreversible pulmonary obstruction which would make the patient unlikely to return to support by pulmonary ventilation.

97. Over a protracted period of chronic lung disease, hypoxia becomes the respiratory drive when the patient accommodates a new higher setpoint of CO_2 tension. If the hypoxia drive is suppressed, ventilatory drive is reduced, and further hypercarbia may result, giving CO_2 tension levels that are anesthetic, dropping respiratory drive altogether. In the acute conditions listed, such as protozoan or bacterial pneumonia or congestive failure, oxygen therapy is a primary indication.

98. Resectability defines the tumor whereas operability is a property of the patient. In this instance we have a tumor that can be resected for surgical excision that is presumably curative in intent for lung cancer, but would further compromise a pulmonary cripple so that life cannot be sustained without — and probably even with — ventilator therapy and oxygen enrichment. This situation represents a tumor that can be resected in a patient that ought not be operated on.

99. An enzyme deficiency is identified with pulmonary emphysema of early onset. Cystic fibrosis or mucoviscidosis is more characteristically associated with bronchiectasis and acetylcysteine is helpful in its treatment. Both tracheoesophageal fistulae and pulmonary agenesis are not conditions associated with pulmonary emphysema of early onset.

100. Any condition that decreases sensitivity toward aspiration response such as suppression of cough reflex with narcotics, obtundation and coma from injury or toxicity predisposes toward gastric contents aspiration, particularly if nausea and vomiting are simultaneously stimulated. A number of infant asthma attacks, particularly those that happen when the patient is supine following eating, are found to be secondary to aspiration. Laryngectomy creates a permanent laryngostomy, and although aspiration of environmental contaminants is possible, gastric aspiration is precluded by this diversion.

101. Prolonged stasis from immobilization with orthopedic or neurologic impairment sets up the conditions whereby lower extremity deep venous thrombosis and embolism may result. Hypercoagulability as with some cancers or viscous blood flow such as polycythemia may allow blood to clot in vessels more readily. Thrombocytopenia makes blood clotting and embolism less likely.

102. Bronchospasm is a condition of smooth muscle contraction constricting the airways, sometimes stimulated by and often made worse by the mechanical action by endotracheal suctioning. To overcome the smooth muscle tonic contraction, bronchodilators may be used that either employ the β-adrenergic effect of catecholamines, or relax smooth musculature directly in muscular blockade paralysis. A specific bronchodilator operating independent of either muscular blockade or catecholamine effect (and useful in instances of bradykinin bronchoconstriction in which catecholamines are contraindicated, such as carcinoid syndrome) is the use of somatostatin analog octreotide.

103. A chest tube is used to evacuate fluid from the pleural space in order to re-expand the residual lung. These fluids could be lymph, blood, or air; however, if the lung on that side of the mediastinum is completely removed, fluid accumulates to form a later fibrothorax, so no tube is used with pneumonectomy.

Items 104-113

104. Infusion of which fluid would be **INAPPROPRIATE** therapy for a patient four hours post 40% full thickness body surface burn?

    (A) Ringer's lactate
    (B) 25% albumin
    (C) packed red blood cells
    (D) plasma
    (E) hetastarch

105. What does the blood type "O+" signify?

    (A) the patient is positive for type "O" antigens on the red cells
    (B) the patient is a universal donor
    (C) the patient is negative for antigens "A" and "B" but positive for rhesus antigen
    (D) a unit of this blood should not be given to a 50 year-old man who is type "AB-" with a negative cross-match
    (E) a unit of this blood should be given to a 5 five year-old girl who is "O-" if the cross-match is negative

106. What percent body surface is burned if a patient is scalded by a spray that strikes the right side of the body circumferentially burning right leg and arm and the torso to the front and back midline, sparing the head and genitalia?

    (A) 18%
    (B) 36%
    (C) 45%
    (D) 63%
    (E) 72%

107. What would be the anticipated mortality if the burn of the extent just described were full thickness in a 40 year-old patient?

    (A) 15%
    (B) 35%
    (C) 45%
    (D) 63%
    (E) 85%

29

108. If crystalloid and colloid are both employed for the support of a 70 kg patient with full thickness 45% body surface burn, what would be the net total volume required in the first 24 hours?

    (A) 3.0 liters
    (B) 5.0 liters
    (C) 6.5 liters
    (D) 8.0 liters
    (E) 10.0 liters

109. As remobilization of the sequestered extracellular fluid takes place, the volume requirements may decrease, but the energy requirements of healing have just begun. For a significant thermal injury as just described, the caloric requirement would approximate a daily total of

    (A) 1000 kcal
    (B) 2000 kcal
    (C) 3000 kcal
    (D) 4000 kcal
    (E) 5000 kcal

110. If 3000 ml of fluid are being given one week post-burn and each contained 5% Dextrose solution, what is the calorie shortfall for the demand that must be made up?

    (A) 600 kcal
    (B) 1000 kcal
    (C) 1500 kcal
    (D) 2400 kcal
    (E) 5000 kcal

111. A patient with closed head injury is not recovering cerebral function when it is discovered that the serum sodium is 88 mEq/L. The appropriate immediate initiation of therapy is

    (A) push an intravenous bolus of 250 ml hypertonic saline solution
    (B) 10% NaCl solution instilled via nasogastric catheter
    (C) furosemide diuresis
    (D) restrict water intake
    (E) insufflate synthetic ADH as a snuff in the nasopharynx

112. Following prolonged aortic cross-clamping, the patient enters the intensive care unit and is found to have cardiac arrhythmia, decreased urine output and a serum potassium of 8.6 mEq/L. Each of the following treatments is appropriate **EXCEPT**:

   (A)   slow infusion of calcium gluceptate
   (B)   set ventilator for hypoventilation and increase respiratory dead space
   (C)   infuse 50% glucose with 10 units regular insulin
   (D)   2 ampules of sodium bicarbonate infused in the arm opposite the calcium infusion
   (E)   potassium exchange resin (kayexalate) by retention enema

113. Eighteen hours post total thyroidectomy the patient is found in carpopedal spasm and complaining of tingling and shortness of breath. Each of the following maneuvers is appropriate **EXCEPT**:

   (A)   rebreathing into a bag
   (B)   infuse calcium gluceptate IV
   (C)   administer mithramycin
   (D)   give large amounts of oral calcium antacid tablets
   (E)   begin vitamin D treatment by mouth

ANSWERS AND TUTORIALS ON ITEMS 104-113

The answers are: **104-C; 105-C; 106-C; 107-E; 108-D; 109-C; 110-D; 111-D; 112-B; 113-C**.

104. The patient within a short period post burn is not likely to be loosing any appreciable quantity of the cellular component of whole blood. However, transudation of plasma and fluid is happening very rapidly following the burn injury, and hemoconcentration is taking place in the patient's circulation. On admission the hematocrit is likely to be rising to levels that are already too viscous for effective circulation, and packed red blood cells would further exacerbate this problem. The patient needs fluid and fast and in high quantities — the most readily available would be crystalloid, and it must be given to replace that which is lost. To maintain a longer period of circulating intravascular fluid, some colloid component of it may be important to sustain circulation, and plasma, albumin, and plasma expanders such as hydroxyethyl starch may serve this purpose. Packed red cells are contraindicated at this stage.

105. The major blood groupings identified the major red cell incompatibilities as based on one antigen or another, both or neither (A, B, AB, O); and to this was later added a minor, but significant incompatibility discovered through transplacental sensitization in succeeding pregnancies found to be present also in the rhesus primate (Rh +/-). This blood type demonstrates neither A nor B antigens with Rh being positive, yet this blood type is by no means universal in that it can be given to anyone. After major antigen typing, it is important to exclude a large number of minor incompatibilities that would lead to hemolysis with over a score known and probably an equal unknown number yet to be fully described, and that is done with a cross-match to rule out presensitization and the presence of preformed hemolytic antibody. That there is no reaction in cross-match might mean that it is worth the risk of Rh sensitization in the middle age man who needs blood, but that may not be the best policy for the young girl whose reproductive future may be compromised since we will not know until the event whether a future fetus might have received the genes that determine Rh positivity in it that will run into potential difficulty with Rh antibody induced by this transfusion sensitization. Major blood group typing, like tissue typing, attempts to minimize sensitization across compatibility differences in specificity, and the cross-match attempts to eliminate hemolytic reaction from preformed antibodies that the donor unit could encounter.

106. The classic "rule of 9's" states that the upper extremity is 9%, the front and back of the torso each 18%, and the lower extremity in entirety 18%, with 9% for the head and 1% for the genitalia. If the patient experienced a burn of half the body (18%), one complete upper extremity (add 9%) and one complete lower extremity (add 18%) the patient has a 45% body surface burn, if the head and genitalia are spared which together are 10% (with corresponding mirror image of the body given the additional 45%).

107. For a full thickness loss of this extent, the age and extent of burn sum to approximate expected mortality. In this 45% full thickness burn in a 40 year-old sums to a high mortality risk of 85% all other factors not considered. If by reason of good health and meticulous surgical care, an extent of burn as described could show satisfactory improvement on those odds with a great deal of energy input.

108. Assuming the patient normally needs 2 liters of water for insensible losses as a daily fluid requirement without the burn, the injury requires the following additional fluid: one-half ml per kg times percent full thickness loss is in colloid (.5 x 70 x 45 = 1575 ml colloid) and three times that in crystalloid (1.5 ml x 70 kg x 45% burn = 4725 ml crystalloid). Adding 2000 ml of D5/W to the 1575 ml colloid and 4725 ml crystalloid sums to 8300 ml total fluid volume, which approximates 8 liters in his first 24 hours post burn.

109. In the absence of infection, just the energy requirement for this degree of thermal injury would be two to three times basal level even given bed-rest. Now that quantity of caloric energy will have to be supplied along with the fluids being given.

110. If the patient's requirements are 3000 kcal and the equivalent of 3000 ml D5/W are being given, the shortfall can be calculated by determining the caloric delivery presently. Since D5/W has 50 gm glucose in a liter, three liters gives 150 grams of glucose. Each gram of glucose supplies four kcal, so (150 x 4 = 600 kcal) are being delivered with a 2400 kcal shortfall. It is unlikely that this will be able to be adequately repleted with the same glucose concentration speeded up, since the volume requirements are no longer as high, so the glucose must be enriched or other energy substrates added. Amino acids have the same value in terms of 4 kcal/gm, but they supply other nutrient needs. Adding some component of lipid doubles the kcal/gm of nutrient value. At one week post-burn, he may be able to take in enriched feedings by mouth. But the maintenance fluid should be shifted now for caloric enrichment whereas the primary requirement early in the post-burn course was for fluid volume and colloid. Over a prolonged period if no return to regular diet of mixed varieties of foods can take place, then trace metals and vitamins must be supplemented. All of this is assuming a normal recovery without intercurrent complication that force up demand and decrease utilization of energy fuels, such as sepsis, which is very likely in a burn of this extent).

111. This patient has severe hyponatremia and it may account for the encephalopathy that persists after his closed head injury. Administration of concentrated sodium by either IV or gastric route may be necessary as may diuresis be, but each is a second order treatment to attempt free water clearance. The simplest and earliest therapy should be to restrict water or any hypotonic fluid intake. In the syndrome of inappropriate ADH secretion (SIADH) the patient is retaining water and diluting the normal serum electrolytes, and the first objective is to keep this from getting worse by additional water intake. Since the ADH activity is excessive, exactly the wrong thing to do is to add additional ADH, which is a treatment for a problem opposite the one that is keeping this patient from waking up.

112. The emergency response is to decrease hyperkalemia. Then reduce excitability of neuromuscular conductivity and contractility. Calcium stabilizes cardiac membranes despite the continuing excess serum potassium, and the next steps are done to drop the high serum potassium by driving it into the intracellular space. Glucose with insulin crosses the membrane surface and expands intracellular space by glycogen deposits which expands the potassium rich intracellular space while the activation of the membrane pump creates a net flux of potassium into the cells. This is in competitive equilibrium with hydrogen ion, and that is the rationale for reducing hydrogen ion concentration to favor potassium transfer intracellularly. That is the therapeutic reason for the bicarbonate infusion, and it is the same reason that hypoventilation and increasing dead space would be contraindicated in this patient, since respiratory acidosis would counteract the effect of bicarbonate infusion, slow intracellular potassium transfer and worsen hyperkalemia.

113. It is the symptoms that are treated rather than the serum calcium numbers, but the patient complaint appears that support to the falling serum calcium will be necessary, so it should be begun until symptoms are relieved and then chronic support taken over by oral supplements. The vitamin D and calcium tablets accomplish the latter role after the IV calcium infusion. The immediate therapy of decreasing the alkalosis that is usually a part of hypocalcemia from the patient's excitement with the discomfort of tetany is effective in rapidly changing the quantity of ionized calcium in competitive equilibrium, since it is the ionized calcium that is the physiologically active component of the diminished total present in the circulation. Rebreathing causes CO_2 increase in the blood and a rise in the hydrogen ion concentration unbinding the calcium carried on serum albumin with competitive antagonism of rising hydrogen ion. The wrong answer is to prevent absorption of calcium into the blood stream, which is the action of mithramycin. This treatment is for hypercalcemia and has no role in the tetany of hypocalcemia.

Items 114-123

114. With respect to hematocrit, at what level is oxygen flow to peripheral tissues optimal?

    (A) 15%
    (B) 25%
    (C) 35%
    (D) 45%
    (E) 55%

115. Which of the following blood products carries minimal risk of viral disease transmission?

    (A) packed red cells
    (B) serum albumin
    (C) factor VIII
    (D) fibrinogen
    (E) platelet concentrate

116. A patient complains of very annoying pain in both shoulders and one side following laparotomy. Physical examination reveals a coin shaped burn over each deltoid area and lateral thigh. The most likely explanation is

    (A) sterile abscess at injection sites
    (B) electrocution entry and exit sites
    (C) improper application of electrocautery grounding pad
    (D) hypersensitivity reaction to adhesive tape
    (E) nummular fixed eruption from medication hypersensitivity

117. During an open technique colonic anastomosis, pencil tip electrocautery activation produces an explosive noise accompanied by a flash of blue flame. Although the patient is not burned, the whole operating team is alarmed. The most likely source is

    (A) alcohol used in the skin prep
    (B) cyclopropane anesthesia
    (C) a short circuit in the spark gap
    (D) methane ignition
    (E) improper grounding lead on the patient

118. A patient is intubated after anesthesia induction and the endotracheal tube fixed with a "bite block" and tape. The patient is then raised to semi-sitting position for skin preparation preceding thyroidectomy for a large right thyroid nodule. During the opening incision, the blood looks dark whereas adequate oximetry readings had been recorded during anesthesia induction. The most likely explanation is

    (A) kinking of the endotracheal tube deviated by the right thyroid mass
    (B) oxygen tank on anesthesia apparatus has run out and intake has not been switched over to auxiliary
    (C) prolonged paralysis secondary to deficiency in acetylcholine metabolism
    (D) advance of the endotracheal tube lumen into the right mainstem bronchus
    (E) malignant hyperthermia

119. Patients with Graves' disease have a higher rate of which of the following complications attributable to anesthesia technique than patients generally?

    (A) dental fractures
    (B) corneal abrasions
    (C) naso-alar cartilage necrosis
    (D) hypotension
    (E) aspiration

120. A 12 year-old boy with abdominal pain is brought to the operating room and anesthesia induced for laparotomy for suspected appendicitis. As the abdomen is scrubbed, the EKG monitor shows the heart is racing and the blood pressure dangerously high. A spot determination of plasma glucose with a chemical strip shows the blood glucose is elevated. A likely source for this crisis is

    (A) ketoacidosis
    (B) anesthetic reaction
    (C) sickle cell crisis
    (D) pheochromocytoma
    (E) malignant hyperthermia

121. Patients with chronic obstructive lung disease have a higher incidence of each of the following intraoperative complications **EXCEPT**:

    (A) bronchospasm
    (B) pneumothorax
    (C) atelectasis
    (D) pulmonary embolism
    (E) pneumonitis

122. A patient has just undergone left pneumonectomy and is returned to the recovery room. Coughing vigorously on awakening, the patient is extubated, but continues to cough and abruptly produces large volumes of dilute blood-tinged sputum as he is gasping for breath. You should immediately

 (A) reopen the incision
 (B) compress the innominate artery against the sternum with a finger inserted through tracheostomy incision
 (C) place the patient in Trendelenburg with the left side down
 (D) sit the patient up in semi-Fowler's position
 (E) perform bronchoscopic lavage

123. A "street person" is admitted for debridement and irrigation with immobilization of an open fracture of the tibia and fibula that he cannot recall how it happened. The operation is performed under spinal anesthesia, and 48 hours postoperatively he becomes very agitated, incoherent, and bizarre in behavior. Immediate check of blood gases shows normal values without hypoxia. The likely diagnosis is

 (A) pulmonary embolism
 (B) acute schizophrenia with psychotic break
 (C) drug dependance
 (D) "ICU syndrome"
 (E) ischemic heart disease

ANSWERS AND TUTORIALS ON ITEMS 114-123

The answers are: **114-C; 115-B; 116-C; 117-D; 118-D; 119-B; 120-D; 121-C; 122-D; 123-C.**

114. Hemoglobin is the chief oxygen carrier of blood. If there are no other rate limiting factors, the higher the hemoglobin, the greater the oxygen carriage capacity. However, hemoglobin is packaged in red cells, and the packed cell mass reflects not only the amount of hemoglobin if the red cells have the normal concentration within them, but also the rate at which blood can flow through capillaries. Many surgeons and more anesthesiologists might be concerned that a hematocrit of 35% was an indication for transfusion; however, the rheology of blood flow through capillaries is actually superior to that seen at the higher hematocrits which carry with them a higher viscosity resisting peripheral capillary perfusion. When hematocrit is very low, although the flow might marginally improve from that seen at hematocrit of 35%, the sacrifice of oxygen capacity means that oxygen delivery is decreased.

115. Human blood donor products carry with them risks of disease transmissibility from malaria through syphilis and hepatitis to HIV and other virions that may result in later development of communicable disease. Each of the subsequent fractionation steps in preparing blood or plasma constituents attempts to both screen and treat the product to minimize transmission risk. This risk is successively minimized but not reduced to zero in production of any of the listed products except albumin.

116. Electrocautery functions through the concentrated intensity at the narrow point of the cautery tip, with the grounding pad giving a much larger surface for that contact and decreased energy transmission for any unit of surface. If this grounding pad is inappropriately placed, has inadequate conductive lubricant applied, or dislodged, the other electrical conduction skinpoints serve as much more concentrated focal grounding points. The EKG leads used in monitoring the patient during this operation have served that capacity, and electrocautery has caused electrical burns at the sites of Einthoven's triangle. Hypersensitivity to tape, drugs, and other allergy would not have this peculiar distribution, and injection site reaction would be subcutaneous rather than a surface burn.

117. Explosive anesthetic agents have been nearly eliminated from contemporary operating rooms in the US, at least, but anesthetic agents are not the only the flammable gas. One agent often suspected but rarely proven is alcohol vapor. Alcohol flammability is much less than other fuels (which is why Indianapolis 500 race cars have eliminated gasoline and are powered by alcohol for the lower probability of ignition in collision) and there would be minimal to no alcohol residual at the time the colon anastomosis is being done late in the operation.

In the first instance, the alcohol applied to the skin would be minimal, and it would vaporize almost immediately after application and would have been long since gone or so dilute as to be even harder to ignite than it has just been noted to be in liquid form. Whether grounded or not, electrical energy is expected to be generated at the cautery tip, and improper setting can give rise to electrical burns, but does not account for the explosion. It is sometimes a surprise to recognize that microbes generate methane in the colon. The quantity of gas produced, particularly with endoscopic insufflation and vigorous bowel preparation prior to operation, can be decompressed when the colon is open and can be ignited by the spark from electrocautery.

118. When an airway is fixed in position when the patient is in a given posture, the alignment of that intubation must be checked again after the patient's position is changed. With flexion, the tube tip may have advanced since it is fixed at the teeth. The ventilation of both sides of the chest is routinely checked following intubation, but should also be checked following repositioning of the patient. "Running out of gas" is a conceivable but unlikely event, and most operating rooms don't run on bottled oxygen alone. Even room air ventilation would not produce desaturation unless the system were closed to ambient ventilation. Cholinesterase deficiency is a possible encounter, but the patient's ventilation is assisted immediately after paralysis is induced for intubation, and it is continued in the event spontaneous ventilation does not resume. Malignant hyperthermia would not give evidence of desaturation as obviously as other signs.

119. Many patients with Graves' disease have exophthalmus associated with this form of hyperthyroidism. Protection of the cornea from overhanging IV tubes, esophageal stethoscopes, electrical stimulators, and a host of electrical monitoring leads draped over the patient's head is the same as for patients being operated on for other causes, but most patients have the eyelids taped to protect the cornea with instillation of methylcellulose drops or antibiotic ointment. This may also be routinely done with patients with Graves' disease, but with less effectiveness if proptosis makes lid retraction and incomplete closure likely. The desiccation that may occur during the period of anesthesia or superficial contacts with the cornea in their protuberant position are more likely in Graves' disease than in other patients. The other complications listed have no unique predisposing factors with Graves' disease, and some are less likely than for the median incidence for all patients in operating rooms.

120. Both anesthesia induction with or without transient hypotension from vasodilatation, and vigorous abdominal massage during abdominal preparation under anesthesia when the patient's abdominal guarding does not limit the rigor of manipulation, have triggered release of catecholamines from an unsuspected pheochromocytoma. The first encounter with an unknown pheochromocytoma in an operating room has high mortality even under contemporary monitoring and support measures, and the best defense is a low threshold for suspicion of this abnormality. It is further increased in likelihood in the combination of both blood glucose and blood pressure elevations as physiologic effects of the catecholamine excess. It is unlikely that either diabetes or sickle cell anemia would be unknown at this age and in this setting, but neither would give this pattern, nor would hyperthermia. Only in the most general sense is this an anesthetic reaction, since it is more a reaction to the manipulation during this experience, and the physiologic effect of such anesthesia second order phenomena, e.g., vasodilation or hypotension, to which it is reactive.

121. Patients with structural derangement of lung structure such as emphysematous blebs or foci of inflammation have a higher rate of pneumonia following operation with typically lower resistance to inocula such as those that may come from intubation or aspiration. Bronchospasm is significantly higher in those patients with any degree of bronchitis, and atelectasis is the most common complication, each from the higher likelihood of inspissated secretions from the prior pulmonary inflammatory conditions. Pulmonary thromboembolism is related to the perfusion side of the lung, and associated with factors that are common to these patients and others of comparable age and disease distribution with no higher incidence in the chronic lung patient, although the consequences of thromboembolism may be more severe in these patients with compromised functional reserves.

122. What is described here is the rare but disastrous circumstance of blow-out of the bronchial stump soon after pneumonectomy. Saline is typically infused into the chest without chest tube drainage to replace the lung with fibrothorax in healing post pneumonectomy. In the course of coughing, the bronchial irritation from this disruption and leak of this pleural fluid is suggested and the coughing also accentuates the blow-out diameter. The patient is flooded with fluid from the open bronchus into the remaining functional lung, and this constitutes, in effect, acute salt water drowning. Accentuating this with further instillation of saline by bronchoscope is obviously not a good idea. A change in the patient's position can be life saving, with the left side down enlisting the help of gravity to slow fluid entry into the airway, and with the head down, drainage of the aspiration fluid is facilitated. The chest should be opened, but under the controlled circumstances of a return to the operating room, where assessment of the bronchial stump and securing it for both air and water tight seal can be reinforced.

123.   The most probable event in a patient who is agitated postoperatively and the first obligation of the clinician is to assure that hypoxemia is not the cause, as it seems not to be in this instance. Both pulmonary embolism and myocardial infarction can give rise to anxiety and agitation in a patient, but they would not account for the timing and symptomatic state with apparently normal oxygen uptake and utilization. Mental illness is very prevalent among patients who are homeless, and this may or may not be characterized by intermittent psychotic episodes. The ICU syndrome is described as a combination of sleep deprivation and a barrage of stimuli in a very anxiety-provoking situation outside the patient's control. There is no evidence that this patient fits this description or that he is even in the ICU. What is worrisome is the circumstance of his original injury. If he were unaware of how it happened, either he was unconscious at the time of this severe injury or forgot it from some lapse immediately afterwards. "Lost" periods of time such as this are often associated with addiction to narcotics or serious bouts of alcoholism, and the patient's current status compatible with withdrawal.

It is also noteworthy in retrospect that there is some difficulty in the anesthetic course of the patient, but spinal anesthesia obviated some of the observations on "drug appetite" noted with induction of general anesthesia, but it may be noteworthy that the patient's postoperative pain would be less likely to be responsive to normal doses of some analgesic agents. The diagnosis could be proven by a challenge with some reversal agents such as nalorphine, but the patient's requirements at this point are to be comforted and treated for his significant local injury as well as his metabolic response to it. There are alternatives to infusions of alcohol or *ad libitum* narcotics, and others may be employed such as the use of minor or major tranquilizers and sedatives, but only while continuing to prove that his agitation is not due to hypoxemia.

An etiologic cause for agitation following an open fracture in any patient, not peculiar to the given clinical description of this patient, might be fat embolism, and this can be checked by examination of stained urine and other clinical evidence, but it is often reflected in respiratory problems and blood gas abnormalities later. Longer term management and rehabilitation for his orthopedic injury is more likely to be successful than for his addiction, but each must be addressed at this time during his hospitalization with precedence given to his addiction.

Items 124-133

124. To cover a surface wound that the surgeon wishes to revise later by sequentially excising portions of it until only primary unwounded skin is closed for the end result, the graft selected would be

   (A) full thickness free graft
   (B) split thickness skin graft
   (C) banked allograft skin
   (D) xenograft
   (E) microvascular composite graft

125. Which of the following techniques would be most appropriate for an immediate release of scar contracture across joint surfaces?

   (A) full thickness pedicle flap
   (B) split thickness skin graft
   (C) myocutaneous composite graft
   (D) skeletal traction for constant tension on joint
   (E) Z-plasty revision

126. The purpose of "meshing" a split thickness skin graft includes each of the following **EXCEPT**:

   (A) it can be expanded to cover much more surface than the size of the original graft donor site
   (B) it allows oxygenation of the granulation bed
   (C) it conforms to the irregular shape of the recipient bed
   (D) it allows serum to ooze without lifting the graft from its attachment to the bed
   (E) it enhances further wound contracture

127. What is the appropriate sequence for the repair of a cleft lip and palate diagnosed at birth for a young male newborn?

   (A) repair of both cleft lip and palate before baby is released from hospital after birth
   (B) repair of cleft lip at 10 weeks, and cleft palate one year later
   (C) repair of cleft palate at one month, and repair of cleft lip at one year
   (D) repair of nasal deformity as soon as possible after birth, cleft lip at one year and cleft palate at puberty
   (E) repair of cleft lip, palate and nasal deformities at one operation just before the child goes to school at age four

128. A young man is seen in the emergency room after a head-on deceleration collision in which he passed through the steering wheel and struck his face against the windshield. The mandible appears intact, but there are fractures bilaterally and in the central compartment of the face whereby the lower face is "floating" in dysjunction from the cranium. This injury is known as

   (A) LeFort I
   (B) LeFort II
   (C) LeFort III
   (D) temporomandibular dysjunction
   (E) Caldwell-Luc maxillary sinus

129. The management of decubitus ulcers ("pressure sores") involves each of the following components **EXCEPT**:

   (A) prevent compression of the ulcerated area by relief of weight-bearing from the site
   (B) maintenance antibiotic therapy
   (C) contouring of the skeletal protrusion by osteotomy
   (D) excision of the ulcer, devitalized facia and inflammation back to bleeding tissue
   (E) restoration of anatomic padding by transfer in of vascularized skin and subcutaneous tissue with or without muscle

130. Each of the following techniques is currently available and recommended for breast reconstruction following mastectomy **EXCEPT**:

   (A) myocutaneous flap using latissimus dorsi
   (B) saline-filled prosthesis
   (C) myocutaneous flap using transverse rectus abdominis (TRAM)
   (D) silicone implant
   (E) myocutaneous flap using gluteus maximus

131. Which of the following factors is most important in minimization of scar formation in closure of an elective surgical incision?

   (A) size of the suture
   (B) number of throws on the suture knot
   (C) dressing technique
   (D) careful tissue handling
   (E) antibiotic irrigation of the wound

132. Intra-arterial injection of illicit drugs by addicts may give rise to serious problems in the hand. These include all of the following **EXCEPT**:

   (A) Volkmann's ischemic contracture
   (B) the "puffy hand syndrome"
   (C) distal digital gangrene
   (D) carpal tunnel syndrome
   (E) gas gangrene of the deep palmar space

133. Which of the following statements is true of a knife laceration of the wrist in a suicide attempt that has severed several tendons, nerves, and the ulnar artery?

   (A) the severance of the flexor digitorum superficialis may be undetected if the profundus is intact
   (B) the ulnar artery ends should be found and re-anastamosed as early as possible in the procedure
   (C) the patient would likely die from exsanguination if not rescued and resuscitated
   (D) if the nerve ends are not found and repaired at the time of acute injury, it will be too late to attempt to find and fix them at a later date
   (E) the patient will be able to oppose the thumb if the median nerve is sectioned at this level

ANSWERS AND TUTORIALS ON ITEMS 124-133

The answers are: **124-B; 125-E; 126-B; 127-B; 128-C; 129-B; 130-D; 131-D; 132-D; 133-A**.

124. One of the putative disadvantages of split thickness skin grafts is that there is an increased secondary contracture rate. That works to the advantage of the therapeutic intent here, in which there is an intent to consecutively decrease the wound size. A microvascular composite graft would in this instance be totally inappropriate, since imported blood supply along with accessory structures beyond surface epithelium is unnecessary and this process is far too complicated for the simple purposes of resurfacing. Full thickness skin graft would be limited in donor sites, and would not be expandable to cover the defect nor would it contract later in the course of progressive shrinkage which is the intent. Allograft "skin" would not take for a period long enough without immunosuppression which is a very high price to pay for a wound closure and eventual elimination. Xenograft would not take at all, but would be used as a biologic dressing, often until a vascularizable graft can be obtained, and if that would be a split thickness skin graft, that could be used here from the start.

125. Scar contracture across joint surfaces may require much more extensive resurfacing than the scar tissue excised, since *contracture* is the nature of the problem that has lost mobility in the joint. The simplest way to release the scar contracture bands that have caused the joint to be drawn up in flexion contracture is to release these scar bands and to reorient the scars so as to not impair motion of the joint. "Z-plasty" involves the geometric incision of the longitudinal contracting band with upper and lower incisions on apposite sides and at angles to the incised scar. The triangular flaps thus created are interposed, thus releasing the contracture.

If split thickness skin graft were used to resurface the scar excised over the contracted joint surface, the recontracture of this joint can be confidently predicted. Full thickness graft would result in less contracture, and myocutaneous flap still less, but each involves the movement of a considerable amount of tissue with a question about limited number of donor sites which would also require closure. Skeletal traction also results in immobility of the joint — in extension rather than flexion, but is unlikely to be successful if the contracting bands are already present, would be painful in their disruption if possible at all, and would not give immediate results. The best method for immediate scar contraction release to restore mobility would be Z-plasty revision; that is triangular flap interposition along the line of contracture.

126. "Meshing" a split thickness skin graft on a grid allows an expansion of 4 to 1 or more surface area coverage than the original split thickness skin graft surface size. Transudation of serum can occur without lifting the graft, but there is little or no advantage in allowing air or enhanced oxygen directly through the interstices. It can be "accordioned" into conformability to irregular recipient beds and facilitates contracture of the surface wound. For these reasons, "meshed" split thickness skin grafts are highly useful for resurfacing burn wounds or other large granulating surfaces.

127. The sequence of repairs in "cleft craft" begins with the cleft lip, and that is usually repaired by the "rule of tens": (a child at ten weeks, ten pounds and ten grams hemoglobin) undergoes repair of cleft lip, and one year later the cleft palate is repaired. After the lip and palate have already been repaired, plastic revision of nasal deformities, such as insufficient columella length, is postponed until puberty.

Clefts in lip and palate have not remarkably interfered with sucking response on the part of the child, and feeding such an infant is remarkably easier than most parents originally envision. Often spoon feeding is begun earlier than usual. In some underdeveloped areas of the world, adult patients with uncorrected clefts may be encountered. They can undergo cleft lip and palate repair, having fully accommodated appearance and speech defects in that interval, sometimes adjustment to the repaired palate and lip is difficult. Before self image has developed, the cleft lip would have been repaired, and just at the time when speech is becoming a very important issue, the palate cleft will be repaired. At the time of heavy concentration on body image in puberty, revisions of columella or vomer deficiency can be undertaken. This sequential repair in "cleft craft" gives the best functional as well as cosmetic results.

128. In the classification of facial fractures, LeFort III fracture represents craniofacial dysjunction. In this instance, the bony skeleton of the face is separated from the rest of the skull and there is a floating dysjunction. LeFort I fracture separates alveolar ridge and palate from the zygoma and nose. LeFort II fractures the nasion so the central triangle of the face is movable. In LeFort III the entire upper jaw, cheek bones, and nose are movable by grasping the upper teeth while holding the skull, with elongation of the face by distraction. Caldwell-Luc is an opening made into the maxillary sinus, and temporomandibular dysjunction would not necessarily involve a fracture at all. LeFort III is the most severe form of facial fracture, involving separation of the suborbital face from the rest of the skull.

129. Relief of pressure on the ulcerated area — the etiology of the pressure sores — is a method helpful in treatment and also prevention of recurrence. This may also involve relief of the pressure from the inside by rongeuring or excising bony prominences, especially when they may be affected by necrosis and osteomyelitis from the ulcer contamination. This means that excision of the devitalized tissue back to bleeding tissue would be an appropriate preparation for a recipient bed to have transferred in some vascularized soft tissue with skin, and most probably associated muscle because of its vascularity exceeding that of subcutaneous fat through some rotation of an anatomic well vascularized but expendable bit of autologous tissue. The pressure ulcer did not begin as a wound infection, and is usually not complicated by any systemic sepsis for which the antibiotics would be indicated. Circulating antibiotics would not be delivered through blood flow to an area of ischemia from pressure so that antibiotics would not be delivered to the site where they would be putatively useful. For that reason, maintenance antibiotics would not have a primary role and only infrequently an adjunctive role, being useful only in treatment of an infection complicating the primary problem of pressure ulceration.

130. Yes, the gluteus maximus is used for this purpose, as are the other myocutaneous flaps from latissimus dorsi or "TRAM" flap using microvascular anastomotic techniques. Saline-filled prosthesis is appropriate, but with any prosthetic graft in this position a fibrous capsular contracture may often occur within an encased and hardened shell that is inappropriate as a breast replacement. Such concerns have reached the level of withdrawal from common use of the silicone prosthetic implant, both for reasons of this encapsulation and for alleged immunologic disorders, so this form of prosthetic breast replacement is not currently recommended.

131. All full thickness incisions in skin heal by scar formation. Minimization of that scar formation is addressed by many factors, including the body position of the skin so wounded, the sharp versus blunt damage to the tissue, prolonged exposure and desiccation, contamination, foreign body presence, tension in proximation and motion of the incision site after closure and dressing. Of these, the single most important factor is careful tissue handling in closure.

The wound is immediately closed by a "plasma glue" which is a transudate and sometimes an exudate of the injured tissue when the integument is broken. It is true that fine suture has less reaction than suture of the smae type but larger caliber, but this factor is part of the technique of gentle tissue handling as are also other considerations such as tension of the closure, and suture technique. The dressing that is applied may involve immobilization as in a plaster splint or supracuticular tension such as adhesive tape "butterfly" closure. Irrigation of the wound is significant in removing foreign body and devitalized cells. The presence or absence of antibiotic is much less important, and can be a negative factor if the chemical reaction of the introduced drugs further damages tissue. Each of the other factors in consideration relate to minimization of further tissue damage as in the first rule of medicine or surgery *"primum non nocere"*.

132. Addicts who have exhausted venous access, or for a special sensation known as the "flash" or "hand tripping", resort to intraarterial injection, since the artery can be located by its pulse when adjacent vessels are obliterated or scarred and impalpable. The excipients may embolize distally giving digital gangrene, and arterial occlusion can give rise to Volkmann's ischemic contracture. The material mixed is often quinine since it has comparable texture to the heroin it is used to dilute, and this sets up the redox potential for anaerobic growth so that gas gangrene is a possible deep palmar space infection that may be a risk to both life and limb.

Carpal tunnel syndrome is the entrapment of the median nerve from compression within the limited space at the volar surface of the wrist, often brought upon patients with prolonged amyloid deposit or repetitive manual stress. It would not be typically associated as a complication of narcotic addict angioaccess.

133. This is an unsuccessful method of suicide, as the patient is now aware, since exsanguination is unlikely, and the ulnar artery need not even be identified for anastomosis, since it is expendable, and there are many more time consuming priorities in the procedure that must follow in repair of this injury. It is true that the flexor superficialis tendon disruption will not be noticed if the profundus is intact, since the patient can still flex the fingers up to the distal phalanx with the action of the deep tendons, and flexor tendon injury in the superficialis system must be searched for to be detected. A very significant injury is the section of the median nerve, and it will receive the most meticulous attention in the repair. It is highly disabling, since the patient will not be able to oppose the thumb, because the recurrent nerve from the median innervation of the thumb comes off distal to the laceration. The repair of the median nerve can be accomplished acutely, or this procedure can be done on a delayed basis with results that will not be impaired by the delay. A great deal of the success of the result is dependant upon rehabilitation directed by the patient, and given the circumstances this may be less than ideal; however, the median nerve should take first priority in attention, the flexor tendons next with the profundus being the highest priority and superficial severed tendons the last options in repair while the ulnar artery is simply ligated.

Items 134-136

Each of the following techniques shown in **Figure 1.1** for employing sutures in closure of skin has indications in surgical practice.

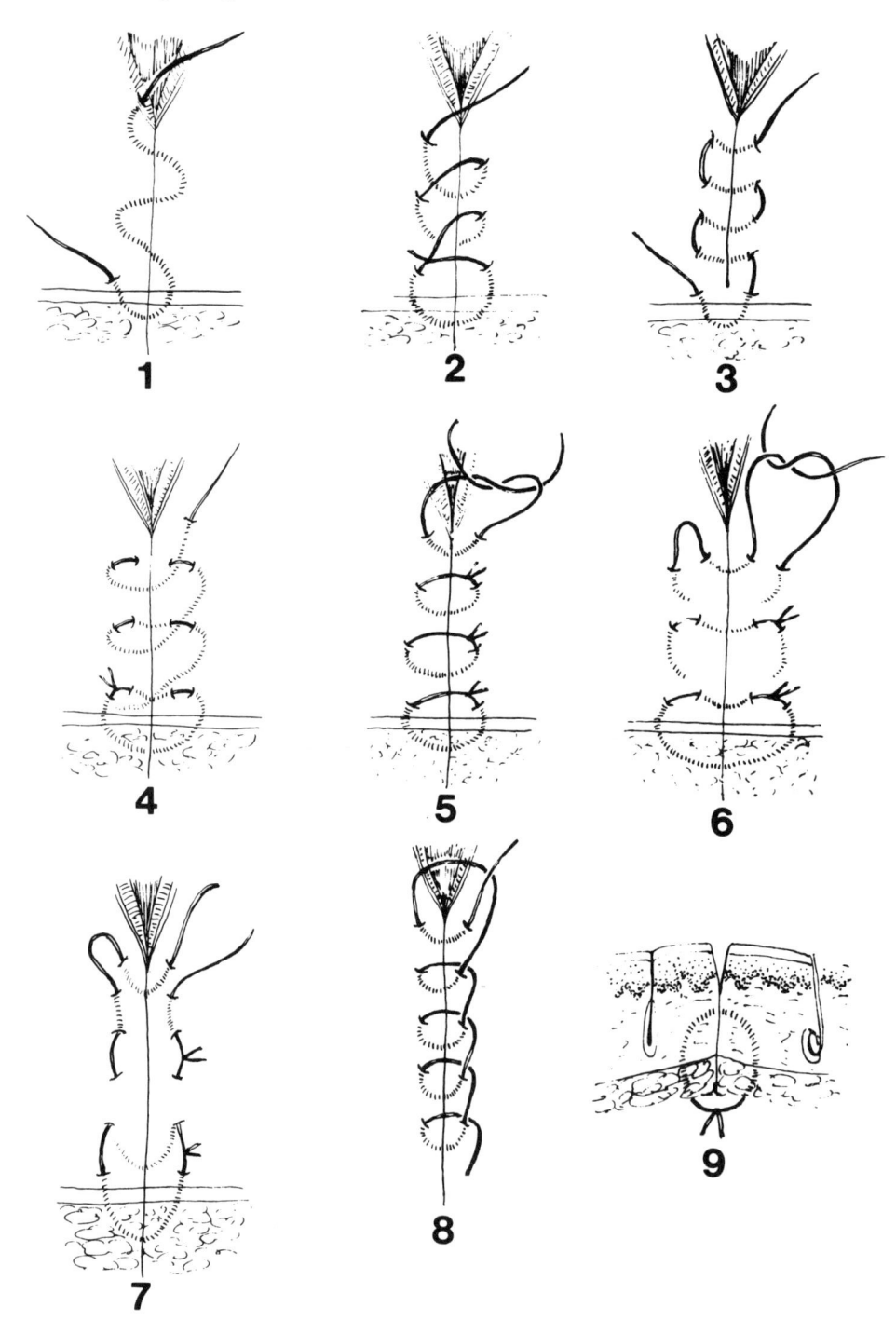

Figure 1.1

134. The interrupted stitch most like to *evert* skin edges.

    (A) 4
    (B) 2
    (C) 5
    (D) 6
    (E) 7

135. The suture **LEAST** likely to leave "stitch marks".

    (A) 1
    (B) 2
    (C) 3
    (D) 4
    (E) 5

136. The suture referred to as "horizontal mattress".

    (A) 4
    (B) 5
    (C) 6
    (D) 7
    (E) 8

ANSWERS AND TUTORIAL ON ITEMS 134-136

The answers are: **134-D; 135-A; 136-D**.

The suture shown in **Figure 1.1**, number 6, above is called the "interrupted vertical mattress". In this technique, the approximated skin edges are everted by the vertical component of the mattress. The suture that is least likely to leave "stitch marks" is one that does not come through the surface of the skin, and in this instance that would be either number 1 or number 9. The number 1 is referred to as the "subcuticular" closure that is continuous, and number 9 is that of an "interrupted buried" subcutaneous suture. The "horizontal mattress" can be either interrupted or continuous as well, but the most common use of this suture is as an interrupted stitch to maintain hemostasis and some compression of the approximated wound edges.

CHAPTER II
ABDOMINAL SURGERY

Items 137-139

This patient complained of symptoms that led to a barium swallow **Figure 2.1A** and then to the finding **Figure 2.1B** seen being repaired in the operating room.

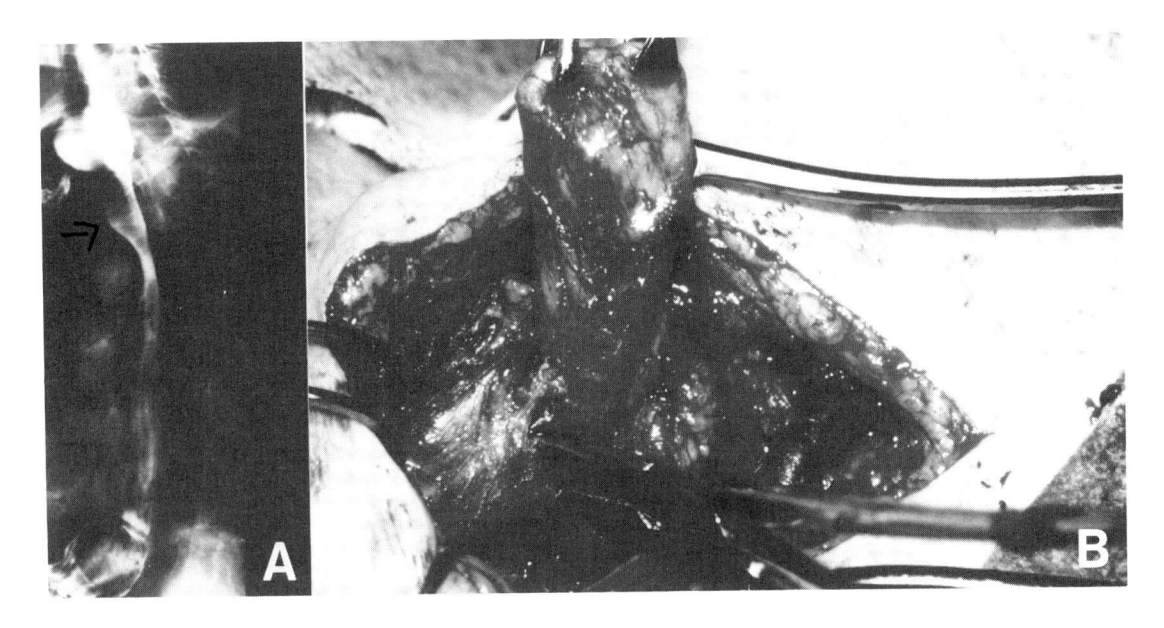

Figure 2.1

137. This finding is most probably

   (A) congenital
   (B) inflammatory
   (C) benign
   (D) malignant
   (E) infectious

138. An etiologic agent is

   (A) lye ingestion
   (B) ionizing radiation
   (C) tuberculosis
   (D) muscular propulsion
   (E) acid reflux

139. Adjunctive to excision will be treatment by

   (A) esophageal bougie dilatation
   (B) myotomy
   (C) corticosteroids
   (D) radiation
   (E) antibiotics

ANSWERS AND TUTORIAL ON ITEMS 137-139

The answers are: **137-C; 138-D; 139-B**.

The specific complaint this patient had when she presented pre-operatively was the regurgitation of food up to several hours after eating that was in no way digested. She said it had also caused her foul breath. The barium swallow shows a Zenker's diverticulum in the classic position. This is a pulsion diverticulum, occurring at the junction of the hypopharynx and esophageal muscles as the decussation allows a mucosal diverticulum to form between the muscular fibers. The diverticulum itself can be either excised, as it was here, or tacked in a position so that it is superior allowing dependant drainage.

Along with the operation to excise the diverticulum is an adjunctive procedure to correct the underlying problem that gave rise to it, and that is by partial myotomy, relieving the constricting pressure that has given rise to the propulsion diverticulum originally.

Items 140-142

A 60 year-old man is referred for evaluation of a distended abdomen shown in **Figure 2.2** with fluid wave and an elevated alpha-fetoprotein. CT shows a large right liver mass.

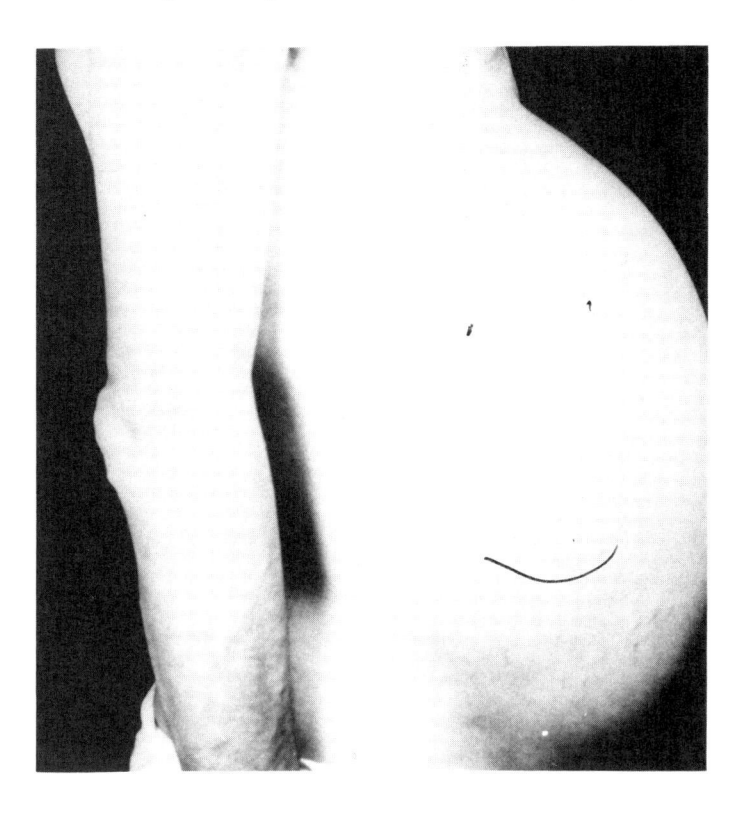

Figure 2.2

140. The patient's operability will be limited by what likely concomitant disease?

    (A) secondary aldosteronism
    (B) Laennec's cirrhosis
    (C) pancreatitis
    (D) congestive heart failure
    (E) renal failure

141. One of the principle determinants of the reserve status that will define operability is

    (A) alpha-fetoprotein
    (B) serum albumin
    (C) Factor VIII
    (D) renal function
    (E) cardiac output

142. Resectability, if the patient is operable, can be facilitated in its determination by

   (A)   ultrasonography
   (B)   hepatic arteriogram
   (C)   cavagram
   (D)   chest X-ray
   (E)   pulmonary function studies

ANSWERS AND TUTORIAL ON ITEMS 140-142

The answers are: **140-B; 141-B; 142-B**.

This patient has the classic clinical appearance of Laennec's cirrhosis. In this instance, the recurrent toxic injury to the hepatic cells has led to continuing scarring, regeneration within a firm and fibrous liver with islands of regenerating nodules. Because the hepatic insult has been metabolic and nutritional rather than focal, the damage is diffuse. For that reason, the estimation of the hepatic reserve will help determine whether the patient is operable. One such measurement that will be critically important is the serum albumin, since the liver is the principle manufacturer of serum albumin as well as prothrombins and other proteins vital for homeostasis and hemostasis. Of these factors, the one most useful in its measurement is the serum albumin.

If it is judged that the patient is operable, the next determination will have to be whether the hepatic tumor is resectable. This determination is often difficult because hepatoma originates in a liver that has underlying cirrhosis. The liver resection can be difficult. Arteriography is useful for determining the extent of spread of tumor and for determining how much hepatic tissue must be resected, and how much viable liver will remain after resection. If the liver resection required would be a trisegmentectomy on the basis of the vascular distribution, and the hepatic reserve is already considerably compromised, the nature of the underlying liver disease and the extent of the primary tumor may combine to make this patient inoperable and the tumor unresectable.

Items 143-145

A 22 year-old woman had a sudden episode of shock brought on by abdominal pain with no antecedent trauma or warning signs. She had been in good health, with her only prior medication being oral progestational contraceptives. She underwent operation with the hepatic findings shown in **Figure 2.3A** and **B**.

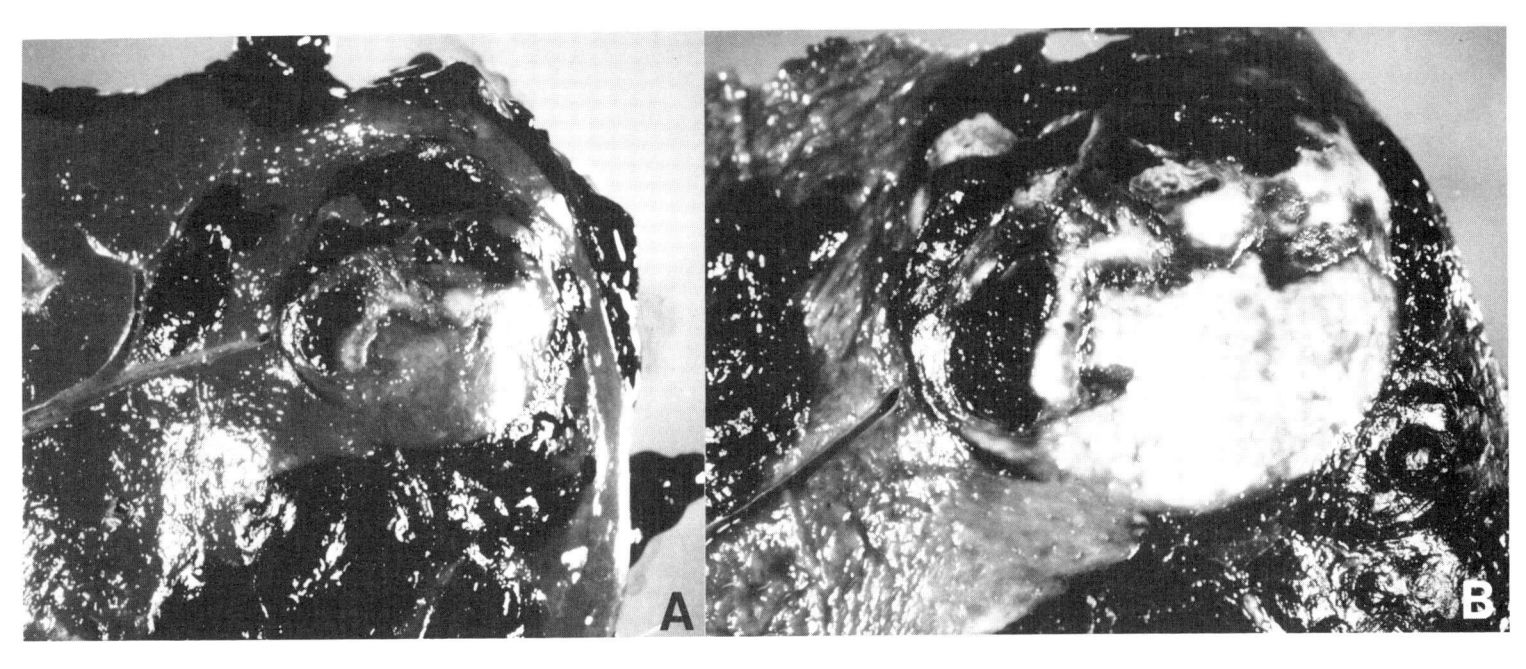

Figure 2.3

143. The tumor type is

    (A) hepatocellular adenoma
    (B) fibrolamellar carcinoma
    (C) cavernous hemangioma
    (D) focal nodular hyperplasia
    (E) angiosarcoma

144. The presentation of this tumor is most often by

    (A) spontaneous hemorrhage
    (B) metastasis
    (C) jaundice
    (D) abdominal mass
    (E) fever of unknown origin

145. The prognosis of the patient after liver resection of the tumor is

    (A)   actuarial
    (B)   limited by toxicity of follow-up chemotherapy
    (C)   dependent on radiosensitivity
    (D)   dependent on presence or absence of estrogen receptors
    (E)   less than 25% 5 year survival

ANSWERS AND TUTORIAL ON ITEMS 143-145

The answers are: **143-A; 144-A; 145-A**.

    This young woman exhibits the classic "pill tumor". The presentation is also classic in that these patients frequently have no antecedent warning before an intra-abdominal hemorrhage brought on by the spontaneous rupture of these benign adenomas. Although they occur infrequently, they seem to occur in the setting of the use of oral contraceptive pills. They closely resemble focal nodular hyperplasia, but those latter tumors rarely rupture, are usually an incidental finding on exploration, and are only weakly associated with the use of oral contraceptives.

    Resection in this instance was for control of bleeding. This having been successfully completed, the patient's survival is actuarial without adverse health impact either on the primary tumor or its treatment. The cell type of the "pill tumor" is that of hepatocellular adenoma.

Items 146-148

A 37 year-old with known lymphoma has an increasing problem with bruising, gingival bleeding and a dropping hematocrit. He undergoes operation with the whole specimen (**Figure 2.4A**) shown and cut section (**Figure 2.4B**).

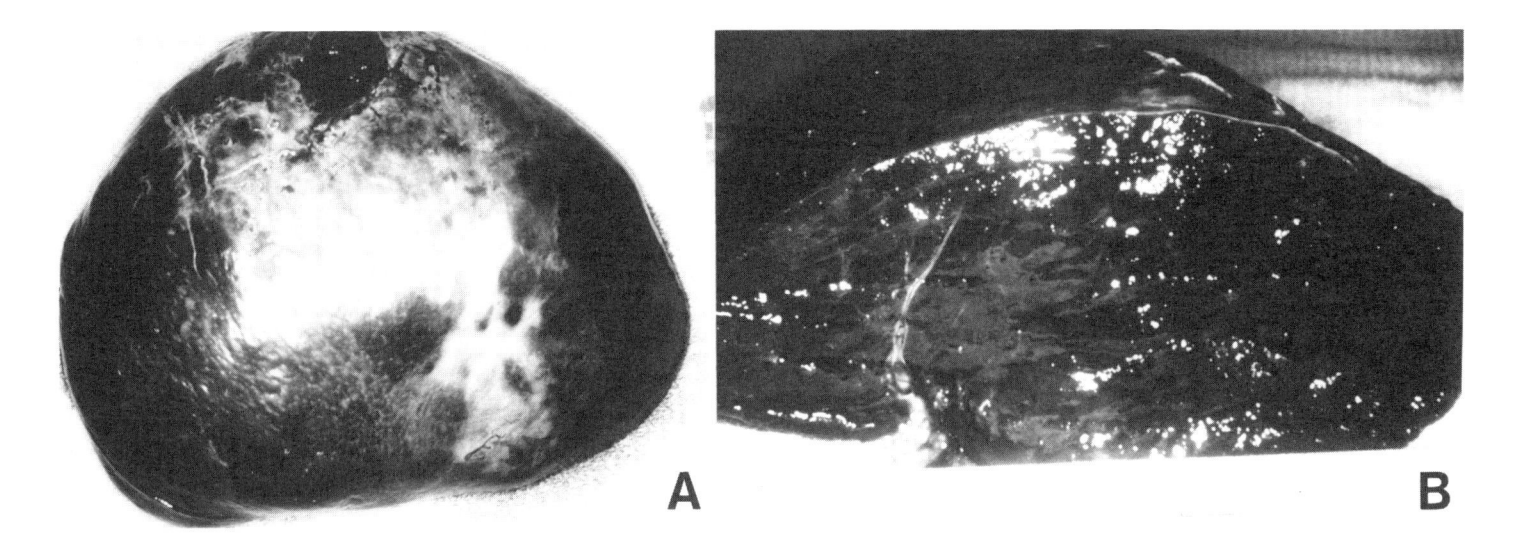

Figure 2.4

146. The indication for operation is

    (A) splenic infarct
    (B) massive splenomegaly
    (C) hypersplenism
    (D) anemia
    (E) pain

147. Platelets administered during operation should be given

    (A) following skin closure in the OR
    (B) one hour after recovery room arrival
    (C) before induction of anesthesia
    (D) at skin incision
    (E) after splenic artery is clamped

148. Left untreated, the biggest risk would be

   (A)　splenic vein thrombosis
   (B)　splenic infarct
   (C)　rupture of the spleen
   (D)　respiratory insufficiency
   (E)　occult (e.g., intracranial) hemorrhage

ANSWERS AND TUTORIAL ON ITEMS 146-148

The answers are: **146-C; 147-E; 148-E**.

This patient has histiocytic lymphoma, and his recent clinical complications are those of hypersplenism. Platelets are very useful as adjunct to operation for hypersplenism, but are most useful when they are given and can remain in the circulation — which they can't be as long as the splenic artery conducts them to splenic filtration out of circulation. Because the single most important feature of hypersplenism in this patient is platelet insufficient in numbers or inadequate in function to prevent spontaneous hemorrhage with minimal or unrecognized trauma, the indication for operation is to reduce this likelihood, since the ease of bruising in the skin surface shows what might be possible in anatomic places where it would do more damage, such as the eye or the central nervous system.

Items 149-151

A 26 year-old woman complains of early satiety and increasing girth. Sonography reveals a startling finding (**Figure 2.5A**), which is followed in 2 weeks by CT (**Figure 2.5B**) after her complaints include abdominal pain. At operation, a mass is found (**Figure 2.5C**), which is sectioned (**Figure 2.5D**)

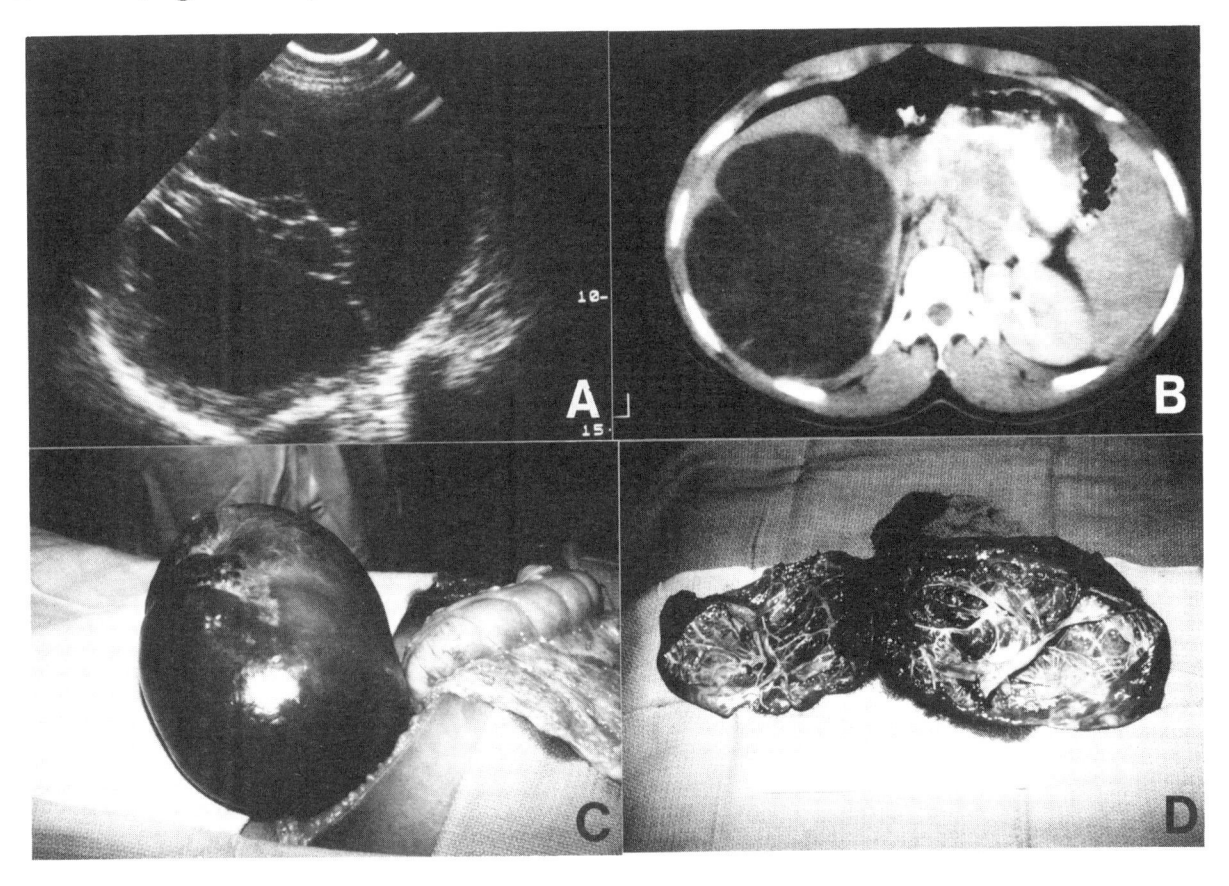

Figure 2.5

149. The likely origin of this lesion is

    (A) hematogenous sepsis
    (B) *Echinococcus granulosus*
    (C) congenital
    (D) hypersplenism
    (E) lymphoma

150. The most likely risk from this finding if untreated would be

    (A) thrombocytopenia
    (B) rupture
    (C) splenic vein thrombosis
    (D) amyloidosis
    (E) pancreatitis

151. This condition under ordinary circumstances is usually

    (A) self limited
    (B) pre-malignant
    (C) an emergency
    (D) associated with portal hypertension
    (E) presenting as sepsis

ANSWERS AND TUTORIAL ON ITEMS 149-151

The answers are: **149-C; 150-B; 151-A**.

This patient has a splenic cyst of amazing dimensions. Not only is it easy to see why her complaints of early satiety have been prominent, it is also easy to see that the most likely event involved in the occurrence of any trauma directed to the abdomen is a rupture of this very large cyst. Most such cysts are self limited, and do not achieve these dimensions. The conditions listed are not related to splenic cysts, which most usually behave in a very benign fashion without causing complication other than a startling finding as on this patient's X-ray and sonography.

Items 152-154

A 51 year-old woman had a colon polyp removed by sigmoidoscopy. The frond-like pattern seen on this section (**Figure 2.6A**) caused concern and a resection of the sigmoid colon was performed with a second polyp seen in micrographic pattern (**Figure 2.6B**).

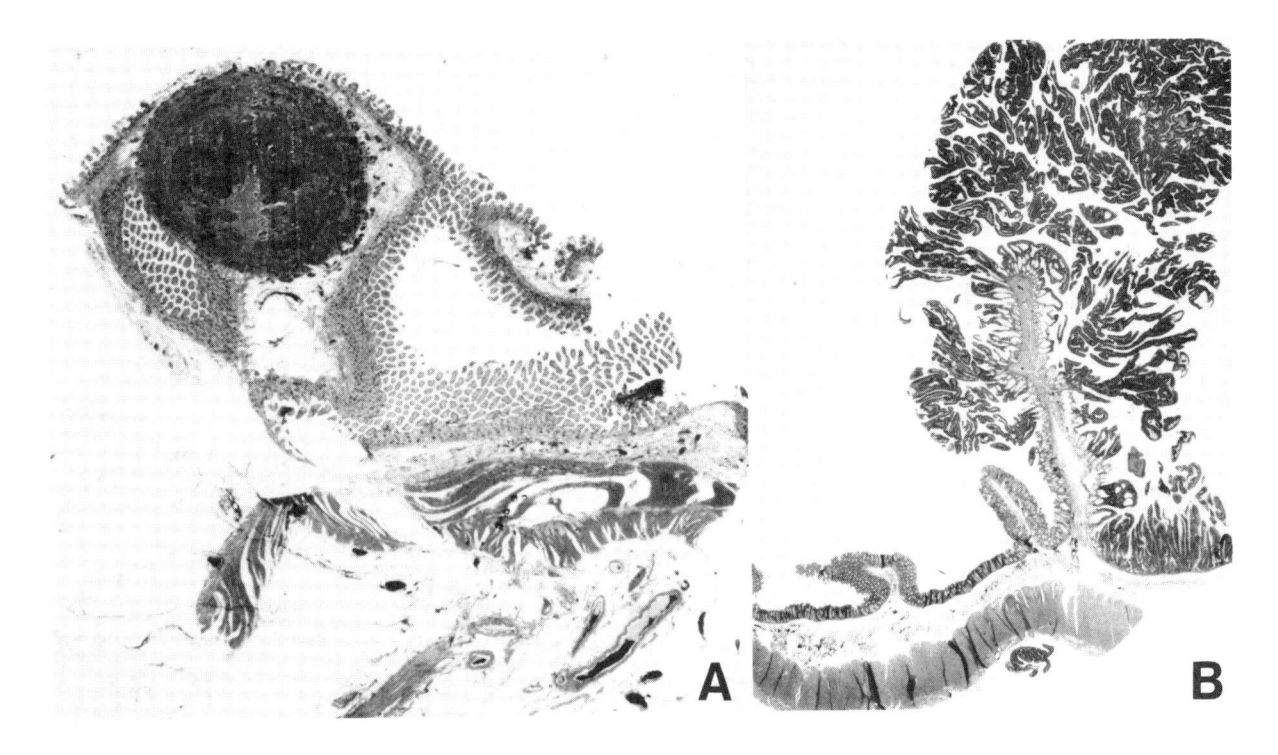

Figure 2.6

152. This appearance is compatible with a diagnosis of

   (A) adenomatous polyp
   (B) villous adenoma
   (C) colonic pseudopolyp
   (D) familial polyposis
   (E) juvenile polyposis

153. The problem for which resection was indicated is

   (A) inadequate margin
   (B) inflammatory potential
   (C) carcinoid
   (D) adenocarcinoma in specimen
   (E) necrotic specimen

154. Following this resection, one would expect her prognosis for 5 year survival to be

    (A) 95%
    (B) 80%
    (C) 60%
    (D) 40%
    (E) 25%

ANSWERS AND TUTORIAL ON ITEMS 152-154

The answers are: **152-B; 153-D; 154-A**.

These life size cut sections of colonic polyps are those of villous adenomata. In the stalk, but not in the base, adenocarcinoma limited to the mucosa and not involving the margins is the indication for the resection of this villous adenoma. No further therapy would be necessary and a very good prognosis would be highly likely for a patient with a disease limited to this minimal origin in a resected villous adenoma.

Items 155-157

After workup for occult blood in the stool, a 54 year-old woman has right hemicolectomy with the specimen shown in **Figure 2.7**. This specimen shows an ulcerative adenocarcinoma with extension through the muscularis mucosae and negative nodes.

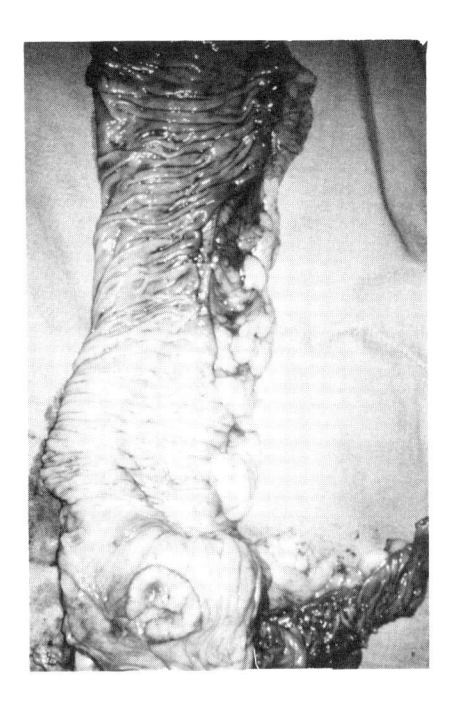

Figure 2.7

155. This would represent Duke's Stage

    (A) A
    (B) B_1
    (C) B_2
    (D) C_1
    (E) D

156. This early detection and treatment for a cecal colon carcinoma would have a 5 year survival prognosis of

    (A) 98%
    (B) 85%
    (C) 60%
    (D) 30%
    (E) 5%

157. Following this treatment, she should undergo serial screening with each of the following **EXCEPT**:

   (A)   CEA determinations
   (B)   stool guaiac
   (C)   liver CT scan
   (D)   colonoscopy
   (E)   digital rectal exam

ANSWERS AND TUTORIAL ON ITEMS 155-157

The answers are: **155-C; 156-B; 157-C**.

A colon adenocarcinoma that extends through the muscularis mucosae as the extent of this local invasion without nodes that are positive represents Duke's Stage B_2. Survival free of disease should be 85% for such a lesion given the treatment of right hemicolectomy. Serial determinations of CEA and a search for a new primary or recurrent tumor using stool guaiac, rectal examination, and colonoscopy would be appropriate, but the liver CT scan would only be done for reason of a positive screen on one of these serial follow-up tests, and would be done for cause of suspicion of such findings and not as a primary follow-up screening method.

Items 158-160

A 48 year-old woman has had diarrhea, muscle weakness, and one episode of lower GI bleeding. A large polypoid mass is found on barium enema examination leading to a sleeve resection of the colon with the polypoid lesion shown in **Figure 2.8** after repeated sigmoidoscopic biopsy was benign.

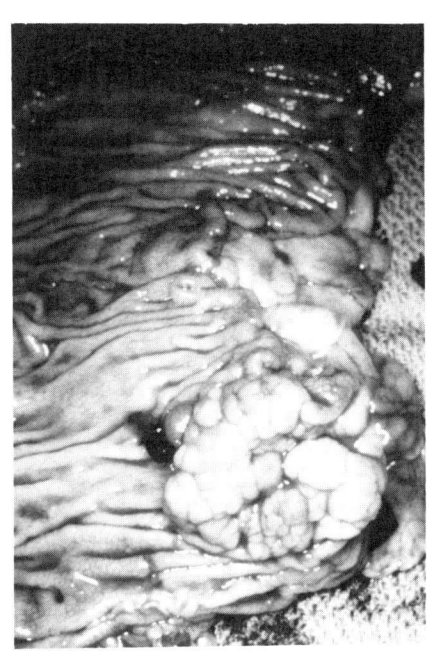

Figure 2.8

158. The history and appearance of such a lesion are most compatible with

    (A) polypoid adenoma
    (B) lymphoma
    (C) villous adenoma
    (D) carcinoid
    (E) leiomyoma

159. Sleeve resection of the colon bearing the polyp was selected as an appropriate operation for each of the following reasons **EXCEPT**:

    (A) lymph node dissection *en bloc* is unnecessary
    (B) standard anatomic colon operations are harder to do
    (C) the lesion is limited to the mucosa
    (D) there is no need for wide margins
    (E) the lesions are not usually multiple

160. The principle reason for removing this lesion is

   (A) premalignant potential
   (B) secretory diarrhea
   (C) tendency to intussusception
   (D) can cause extensive hemorrhage
   (E) recurrence

ANSWERS AND TUTORIAL ON ITEMS 158-160

The answers are: **158-C; 159-B; 160-A**.

This patient exhibits a large villous adenoma with a characteristic clinical history leading to its discovery by both barium enema and sigmoidoscopic examination. Repeated biopsies showed no malignant degeneration, but endoscopic removal was not possible because of its size and pedicle. Because this is a benign lesion, the colon bearing this lesion was resected by a sleeve resection rather than a standard anatomic colon procedure which is designed to encompass the venous and lymphatic drainage of the lesion, unnecessary in this case because there would be little likelihood of metastatic potential from a benign lesion. No wide margins are needed and the lesions are not typically multiple, so this was a conservative colon resection for a large lesion that was not only symptomatic, but also has a high degree of malignant potential, and consequently operation is indicated. The operation for any benign colon polyp is different from that for a malignant tumor of the colon when that is confidently predicted pre-operatively as it was in this instance; otherwise, a standard colon operation as for adenocarcinoma would be appropriate if the nature of the lesion were indeterminate.

Items 161-163

This barium swallow in **Figure 2.9** was ordered to evaluate the condition of a patient with symptoms of hiatal hernia.

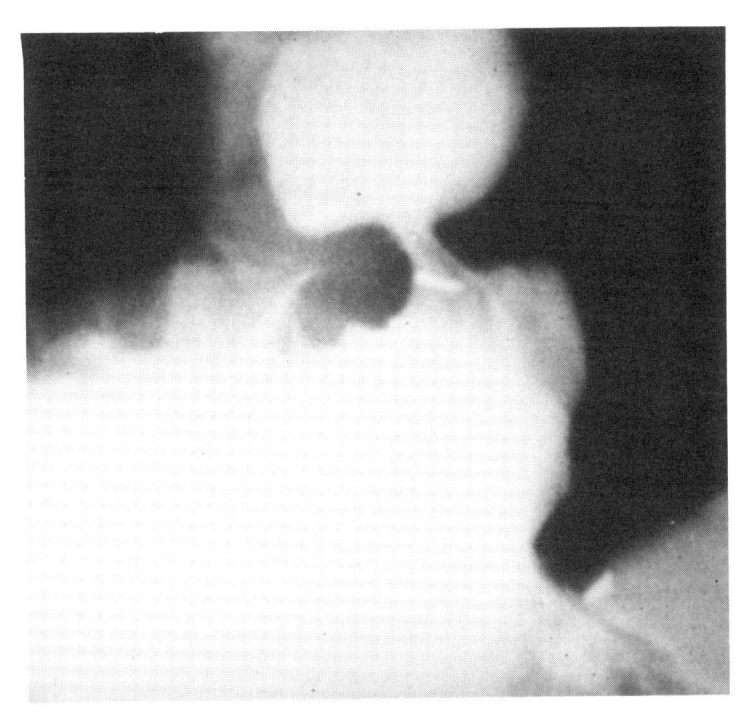

Figure 2.9

161. The lesion demonstrated is probably

   (A) congenital
   (B) inflammatory
   (C) malignant
   (D) not serious
   (E) responsive to radiation

162. Treatment of this condition employs each of the following **EXCEPT**:

   (A) H_2-receptor antagonists
   (B) operation
   (C) endoscopy
   (D) radiation
   (E) bouginage

163. The therapy will have to include a plan to

   (A)   replace the esophagus
   (B)   pull the stomach up into the chest
   (C)   control systemic spread of disease
   (D)   prevent acid reflux
   (E)   achieve wide margins around the disease

ANSWERS AND TUTORIAL ON ITEMS 161-163

The answers are: **161-B; 162-D; 163-D**.

This patient has esophageal stricture from acid reflux peptic esophagitis. The stenosis is the indication for operation, but simultaneously, some method to prevent acid reflux should take place to minimize recurrence. In this instance, that can be surgical if there will be a surgical treatment for the stenosis, but medical therapy is often employed as adjunct to or in place of operation for the hyperacidity. That includes each of the options listed with the exception of radiation, which would not be appropriate for a benign condition and would cause further fibrotic stenosis.

Items 164-167

    (A)   Cholecystitis
    (B)   Cholangitis
    (C)   Both
    (D)   Neither

164. jaundice

165. stones

166. mortality

167. sphincteroplasty

ANSWERS AND TUTORIAL ON ITEMS 164-167

The answers are: **164-B; 165-C; 166-B; 167-B**.

Cholecystitis is a disease of significant morbidity; cholangitis is associated with high mortality. Both may be associated with gall stones and usually are. Frequently gall stones previously associated with cholecystitis may pass into the common duct producing obstruction and cholangitis. It is this obstructive component of cholangitis that produces the jaundice, which should not be associated with cholecystitis unless cholangitis is involved.

Sphincteroplasty is a method to increase flow and reduce pressure in the common duct, and this release of obstruction of the common duct should relieve cholangitis, but should have nothing to do with the gall bladder, which has its own distal resistance in the spiral valve in the cystic duct at the junction with the common duct. Sphincteroplasty should not relieve cholecystitis, although it is a method of managing cholangitis. Sphincteroplasty can also allow reflux from the duodenum or pancreatic juices into the common duct, and may therefore be associated with cholangitis as an etiology, but this should be a much more benign condition following sphincteroplasty than that which could occur in its absence in which the inflammation under pressure in the obstructed duct would have a much greater likelihood of going on to septicemia in the patient with obstructed cholangitis.

Items 168-171

        (A)   Hepatitis
        (B)   Hepatoma
        (C)   Both
        (D)   Neither

168. B viral antigen

169. cirrhosis

170. aflatoxin

171. most probably lethal

ANSWERS AND TUTORIAL ON ITEMS 168-171

The answers are: **168-C; 169-C; 170-B; 171-B**.

    Hepatitis B is clearly associated with hepatitis B viral antigen, but so is hepatoma which is the most common lethal visceral cancer in the world, distributed with highest incidence in the regions where the highest serum antibody positivity to the hepatitis B antigen prevails. There is a study in the railway workers in Taiwan that have been followed over twenty years, and it has been found that there may be benefit to hepatitis B vaccination not only in preventing the inflammatory component of hepatitis, but also reducing the incidence of hepatoma which appears to be a late complication of hepatitis.

    Cirrhosis is associated with both hepatitis and hepatoma, since nearly all hepatomas arise in cirrhotic livers, most of which are in the context of hepatitis B seropositivity and having had hepatitis. There have been allegations that aflatoxin is associated with hepatoma, not yet disproved, but overshadowed by the much more powerful evidence of hepatitis B viral etiology for hepatoma as well as hepatitis. It remains a brutal fact that the most common visceral cancer occurs in the parts of the world where the expensive and highly intensive surgical care would be most needed but is least likely to be obtained. It is an even more sobering fact that the surgical treatment is most likely ineffective in either development setting.

Items 172-175

      (A) Chronic pancreatitis
      (B) Pancreatic cancer
      (C) Both
      (D) Neither

172. jaundice

173. surgical cure

174. alcoholism

175. normal serum amylase likely

ANSWERS AND TUTORIAL ON ITEMS 172-175

The answers are: **172-C; 173-D; 174-A; 175-C**.

Both chronic pancreatitis and pancreatic cancer may produce jaundice, and do so with about even likelihood. The classic pancreatic adenocarcinoma that presents with obstruction to the bile duct in the head of the pancreas may represent the only fortunate early presentation because of the location of the disease in the peri-ampullary area. Chronic pancreatitis with peri-ampullary inflammation, alkaline reflux ("common channel") and pseudocyst formation may give rise to obstruction and jaundice with the same frequency as pancreatic cancer arising anywhere in the pancreas does, including those few that obstruct early in the peri-ampullary area.

Alcoholism is a nearly invariable association of chronic pancreatitis but is not remarkable for pancreatic cancer. In both instances the serum amylase is likely to be normal. There may be a higher urinary amylase clearance with pancreatitis, but many of the pancreatic cancers are associated with pancreatic ductal obstruction and some degree of regional pancreatitis, and have as high a likelihood of showing elevations of amylase. In both instances, the most probable serum amylase would be within normal range.

In nearly all instances in which it is employed, surgical therapy is palliative for both conditions. The objective of surgical treatment is typically management of pain, diversion of obstruction of gastric outlet or bile flow, and minimizing disruption of gastrointestinal function. That does not mean that radical operations are not undertaken with intent to cure, but the somber fact remains that the majority of those curative attempts are futile and proven so with distressingly frequent failed postoperative results.

Items 176-179

(A) Benign gastric ulcer
(B) Malignant gastric ulcer
(C) Both
(D) Neither

176. treatment with H_2-receptor antagonists

177. associated microorganism

178. pernicious anemia

179. elevated gastrin

ANSWERS AND TUTORIAL ON ITEMS 176-179

The answers are: **176-A; 177-A; 178-B; 179-A**.

Gastric ulcers have a difference in distribution in the stomach and differing etiologies. With peptic ulceration, there is a bacterium (*Helicobacter pylori*) implicated in loose association with some suggestion that benign peptic ulcer could be an infectious disease. This organism is associated with peptic ulceration so that it would be the benign gastric ulcer. Gastric malignancy is associated with hypochlorhydria. This hypochlorhydria and atrophic gastritis are often features of pernicious anemia. Because malignant gastric ulcers already occur in a state of decreased gastric acidity, H_2-receptor antagonists would not be appropriate as treatment. Whereas the cephalic phase of gastric acid stimulation is very prominent in duodenal ulcer, gastrin elevation is a principle stimulus to HCl production in benign gastric ulcer with its associated high acidity, not the response seen in the event of the low acidity of the malignant gastric ulcer.

Items 180-183

        (A) Esophagitis
        (B) Esophageal cancer
        (C) Both
        (D) Neither

180. stricture prominent

181. perforation a significant concern

182. surgical cure

183. colonic interposition

ANSWERS AND TUTORIAL ON ITEMS 180-183

The answers are: **180-C; 181-C; 182-A; 183-C**.

Esophagitis and esophageal carcinoma both have esophageal stricture as a prominent part of their presentation and this represents a continuing patient management problem. Perforation is a very prominent possibility for both, especially since each is diagnosed, biopsied, and observed with semi-rigid endoscopes. Both consist of friable tissue and neither have any serosa to contain any mucosal penetration that erodes muscle. Therefore, for both conditions, perforation is a significant concern.

Surgical treatment is employed for each of these conditions, although medical therapy is primarily indicated for esophagitis. Surgical treatment may be indicated if medical therapy does not control the disease. The esophageal carcinoma is not treated medically, but surgical attention is directed toward relief of obstruction, and only in rare instances is resection for curative rather than palliative intent appropriate. Whereas there are many procedures to correct reflux esophagitis, and many of them have the satisfying result of surgical cure, most prominent among these surgical procedures being the Nissen fundoplication, surgical cure is a fatuous hope for the vast majority of patients with esophageal carcinoma of the stage it typically is at presentation. Surgical treatment has such a high probability of failure in curative intent that it should principally concentrate on its palliative role. In contrast, there is a significant probability that the patient with esophagitis might be cured if antireflux operations are performed.

Colonic interposition replacement of the esophagus is necessary in some instances when very high resection of the esophagus is necessary for esophageal carcinoma and the more common procedure of the pull-up of the stomach into the chest is thought inappropriate. Colonic interposition is also indicated for some forms of esophagitis, especially following multiple complicated and recurrent procedures for esophageal stenosis of significant segmental length, and many of those that involve lye ingestion and the extensive destruction of the esophagus that this form of esophagitis entails.

Items 184-188

    (A)   Hepatitis
    (B)   Cirrhosis
    (C)   Cholecystitis
    (D)   Peri-hepatitis (Curtis-Fitzhugh)
    (E)   Cholangitis
    (F)   Portal vein thrombosis
    (G)   Hepatoma
    (H)   Hypersplenism

184. *Gonococcus* is an etiologic factor.

185. Obstructive jaundice often associated.

186. Associated with abrupt onset of varices.

187. Three-fold elevation in alpha-fetoprotein (AFP).

188. *Salmonella* carrier state.

ANSWERS AND TUTORIAL ON ITEMS 184-188

The answers are: **184-D; 185-E; 186-F; 187-G; 188-C**.

Pain over the liver may not be due to a problem originating in the liver. That is the case with pelvic inflammatory disease, which can give pericapsular adhesions which are related to the same pelvic inflammatory process and its etiologic agents. The early causes of pelvic inflammatory disease include *Gonococcus*, but later, a variety of organisms may be responsible for the Curtis-Fitzhugh syndrome, particularly if the origin is from chronically scarred adnexa with repeated antibiotic therapy changing the flora.

Cholecystitis is a condition of some morbidity, but may be asymptomatic, and resident parasites may be lodged in the gall bladder in the chronic carrier state for such patients as can spread typhoid. *Salmonella* has a propensity for the biliary tract as a residence in the carrier state.

In contrast to cholecystitis morbidity, cholangitis is a disease of high mortality, and that risk is often related to not only the sepsis associated with it, but also the obstruction potential in which the bile necessary for both liver excretion and secretion cannot achieve access to the gut. Therefore, inflammation in the biliary tree, as distinct from the parenchymal hepatocytes, with jaundice, suggests obstruction of the common bile duct rather than simply the cystic duct.

Cirrhosis can give rise to esophageal varices, but that typically takes place over a prolonged period of time, and may be infrequently abrupt in onset or at least recognition. However, a source of acute portal hypertension is portal vein thrombosis. This may be secondary to extension from the mesenteric venous drainage of the gut, and that may be due to inflammatory processes or obstructive phenomena within the GI tract. In cirrhosis and hepatitis there is occasionally an elevation in the AFP, but when that elevation becomes quite significantly greater than normal, hepatoma is a likely source of excess values in these three-fold ranges.

Items 189-193

GI bleeding from:

- (A) Esophageal varices
- (B) Esophagitis
- (C) Barrett's ulcer
- (D) Mallory-Weiss tear
- (E) Esophageal cancer
- (F) Gastric ulcer
- (G) Erosive gastritis
- (H) Gastric cancer
- (I) Duodenal ulcer
- (J) Hemobilia
- (K) Bleeding Meckel's diverticulum
- (L) Enteritis
- (M) Diverticulosis
- (N) Ulcerative colitis
- (O) Colon cancer
- (P) *Fissure-in-ano*
- (Q) A-V malformations
- (R) Angiodysplasia
- (S) Fistula from arterial prosthetic graft

189. Associated with deceleration liver trauma.

190. Tenesmus.

191. Prolonged vomiting.

192. Most common source of occult blood loss in 65 year-olds in the United States.

193. Balloon compression therapy.

ANSWERS AND TUTORIAL ON ITEMS 189-193

The answers are: **189-J; 190-P; 191-D; 192-O; 193-A**.

Each of the sources listed is a potential site of gastrointestinal tract bleeding. One is peculiar to liver injury, in particular of the kind that leaves a large intrahepatic hematoma, and that is blood decompression into the biliary tree, or "hemobilia". One is characteristically associated with prolonged vomiting, although any may cause vomiting from the irritation of blood in the gastrointestinal tract. However, the one that is associated with prolonged vomiting as an etiologic agent is the Mallory-Weiss tear in the upper gastrointestinal tract.

Esophageal varices, and to a lesser extent those in the epigastric cardia, are treated by tamponade with a compression balloon since the pressure within the varices that is the driving force of the hemorrhage through the ulcerated surface is an elevated portal venous pressure. The balloon would be much less effective if it were designed to stop arterial pressure, since it would not only be unlikely to accomplish that, but if it did it would cause necrosis of the epithelium and further hemorrhage. The one form of lower anorectal bleeding that is highly symptomatic is that of *fissure-in-ano*, which can occasionally give the involuntary spasm of the voluntary muscles known as tenesmus, a highly symptomatic condition. In terms of occult blood loss into the gastrointestinal tract, it is important to remember that benign conditions are less significant than malignancy, and colo-rectal cancer remains the most likely origin of occult blood loss into the gastrointestinal tract in older people in the United States.

Items 194-198

(A) Stress ulcer
(B) Cushing's ulcer
(C) Curling's ulcer
(D) Steroid ulcer

194. Infected ulcers.

195. Closed head injury.

196. Highest mortality.

197. Ablated by vagotomy.

198. Prevented in the ICU by strict neutralization of gastric acid.

ANSWERS AND TUTORIAL ON ITEMS 194-198

The answers are: **194-C; 195-B; 196-A; 197-B; 198-A.**

Secondary ulceration of the upper gastrointestinal tract has been associated with several kinds of critical illness. One of these kinds was described by Curling in patients with severe burns. These patients who have burns and developed upper GI bleeding are found to have peptic ulcer, but only if the patients are infected, as most of the patients with major burns inevitably are.

75

The very ulcers themselves are infected with the same agent that can be cultured from the blood of the burn patient.

The ulcer described by Harvey Cushing is related to an increase in intracranial pressure, which occasioned severe upper gastrointestinal bleeding in a sequential series of sixteen patients. He made the pre-operative diagnosis in the next one in this long series of patients who had undergone intracranial operations with increasing intracranial pressure as the common feature. This is due to strong vagal stimulation which increases acid output, and is therefore interruptable by vagotomy. Since the cephalic phase can be blocked pharmacologically now through antihistamine interception, this would constitute the equivalent of a medical vagotomy with respect to inhibition of gastric acid stimulation.

Stress ulceration is seen with a variety of causes that lead to multiple sequential organ failure, sepsis prominent among them. This is a reflection of the low flow state and an erosion with serpentiginous undermining of the mucosa and diffuse bleeding. Because of the underlying circumstances that give rise to the disease, the mortality is highest among patients with stress ulcer, but the ulceration itself can be minimized by compulsive attention to gastric juice and its neutralization. This can be done by a nasogastric tube with continual titration of the pH to maintain it in excess of 7, or, by a less labor-intensive method, an antihistamine can be given that would block the H_2 receptors and maintain a gastric juice in neutral range with either buffers or receptor blockade.

Items 199-203

(A) Oral cholecystogram
(B) Ultrasound
(C) Harrey-technetium-99m iminodiacetic acid (^{99m}Tc HIDA) scan
(D) CT scan
(E) Hepatic arteriogram
(F) Spleno-portography
(G) Percutaneous transhepatic cholangiogram
(H) Endoscopic retrograde pancreatic cholangiography

199. Acute right upper quadrant pain in a 42 year-old obese woman who has had abrupt pain onset 2 hours after eating.

200. A jaundiced 58 year-old man with pre-operative elevated pancreatic and hepatic enzymes who has failed earlier CT demonstration of abdominal pathology except to show dilated ducts and a portal fullness.

201. An 18 year-old member of a spherocytosis family has had episodes of colicky pain and splenectomy has been considered for persistent anemia.

202. A patient with known cirrhosis and CT-demonstrated large liver tumor is being evaluated as a candidate for operation.

203. A woman with painless jaundice who had a vague fullness found by CT in the peri-ampullary area is being evaluated as a candidate for operation.

ANSWERS AND TUTORIAL ON ITEMS 199-203

The answers are: **199-B; 200-G; 201-C; 202-E; 203-H.**

The typical candidate for acute cholecystitis might have the first study be the last one if ultrasound shows a "halo" of edema around the gall bladder which may be distended and as a bonus, shows gall stones. These gall stones are unlikely to be radio-opaque, so there would be no benefit in getting a flat abdominal film for this relative unlikelihood, whereas the ultrasound has a very high likelihood of achieving a diagnosis sufficient for recommendation of therapy. The ultrasound would also not be limited by a certain level of bilirubin for function, as would both oral cholecystogram and ^{99m}Tc HIDA scan. The ^{99m}Tc HIDA scan would be helpful in the definition of the abdominal pain in the young man with spherocytosis, since the pigment stones are often associated with the gall bladder with enough absorption capacity to still give visualization, and it is faster and more reliable than the oral cholecystogram. A reasonable question might be whether any diagnostic testing was necessary, since the gall bladder might be removed on the basis of the high likelihood that cholecystitis is present and would be, given his underlying hereditary disease, and the likelihood that cholecystectomy could be performed as accessory to an operation already being considered in abdominal exploration.

The other three patients have longer standing liver disease, two of whom have jaundice ruling out tests sensitive to a functioning liver and absorbent gall bladder (oral cholecystogram and ^{99m}Tc HIDA scan). CT scan has already been performed in each of the three which was sensitive to the degree that CT discrimination would be higher than that of ultrasound, but no definite localization of a mass was obtained. In one instance, because of the obstructive jaundice and dilated ducts, the patient is anticipating an operation, and pre-operative percutaneous cholangiography may not only help demonstrate the site of the lesion, but allow pre-operative drainage for better anesthetic and postoperative management in this patient.

In the woman with painless jaundice, peri-ampullary malignancy is anticipated, and an effective way to study this would be with an endoscopic retrograde pancreatic cholangiography. This might not only identify the site of obstruction, but also retrieve tissue for its diagnosis to compare with that seen on the imaging. The imaging studies may indicate operation because of the location of this obstruction (which would include planning both palliative and curative operation) or on the basis of demonstrated extension of the disease that would contraindicate curative resection and recommend limiting the operative strategy to palliation.

One patient already has CT demonstration of a large liver tumor, and at this point, the diagnosis is not the question but the extent of the resection that would be necessary to encompass the tumor and still leave viable amounts of liver. Because there is parenchymal damage from an underlying cirrhosis, it is important to see if this tumor can be resected without the loss of a large majority of the liver or interference with its arterial supply — which is the same thing. If more than 20 to 25% of the liver can be anticipated to be residual with an intact arterial supply not encased by the hepatoma, then curative operation is possible. These studies not only may contribute to diagnosis, but also define resectability and even in some instances help in the determination of operability.

Items 204-208

(A) Upper GI barium swallow
(B) Esophageal gastroduodenoscopy
(C) CT scan
(D) Arteriography

204. A woman suspected of bleeding varices has which primary diagnostic/treatment method of first choosing?

205. After failed sclerotherapy, bleeding rate increases; the next step before operation might be?

206. Which of these tests might still be likely to find the bleeding point if the vessel were bleeding 5 ml/10 min?

207. Which of these tests might demonstrate a small leak in an esophageal anastomosis?

208. Which of these studies may be useful to decrease portal perfusion pressure?

ANSWERS AND TUTORIAL ON ITEMS 204-208

The answers are: **204-B; 205-D; 206-B; 207-A; 208-D**.

Upper gastrointestinal endoscopy is highly specific in diagnosis, and sometimes can be extended to therapy through such means as sclerotherapy in the case of bleeding varices. If the sclerotherapy fails, even when repeated, and if the bleeding rate increases, the next therapeutic step might be arteriography, since pharmacotherapy can be infused through the arteriography catheter to diminish portal pressure through decreasing splanchnic blood flow. When blood flow is minimal, arteriography is not very helpful as a localization method, but minimal blood loss can be detected by endoscopy, even in finding areas where bleeding had been issuing but now was no longer actively bleeding from identification of the ulcerated site.

Both arteriography and CT would not be very helpful in finding the site of a leak, which can often be missed on endoscopy as well. Further, in a fresh anastomosis, there would be no enthusiasm for inserting a fiber-optic tube into a recently postoperative patient, since the anastomotic perforation might be found by causing it. Contrast swallow might be the best way to determine a leak in an esophageal suture line. It is preferred that this be with water-soluble contrast if it is anticipated that it might find its way into the mediastinum, but a recent anastomosis will likely still have chest tubes available, and probably would require re-operation if it were substantial, so a higher definition possible with the greater opacity of barium may be preferable.

Items 209-213

GI bleeding clinical characteristics:

(A) Exsanguinating hemorrhage - patient comes to ER in shock, after 3 units rapid transfusion, patient remains in shock
(B) Severe - the patient comes to the ER in shock, after 3 units of rapid transfusion is no longer in shock, but still actively bleeding
(C) Moderate - patient comes in to ER with evident bleeding, not in shock, but is treated for the bleeding and the bleeding stops, but then restarts, often repeatedly
(D) Occult - evidence of blood loss is an incidental finding, sometime on incidental stool guaiac performed on rectal exam specimen

209. Presenting feature is usually anemia.

210. Bleeding colonic diverticulosis's usual pattern.

211. Requires treatment *before* diagnostic procedures such as X-ray or endoscopy.

212. Upper GI endoscopy preferred diagnostic method.

213. Barium enema is appropriate primary diagnostic procedure.

ANSWERS AND TUTORIAL ON ITEMS 209-213

The answers are: **209-D; 210-C; 211-A; 212-B; 213-D**.

The patient who is experiencing exsanguinating hemorrhage needs therapy, and quickly. This means that there will be no trip to the X-ray suite, nor time for refined diagnostic localization when the patient needs to be resuscitated from shock. This means the patient goes directly from the emergency room to the operating room while intensive support continues in order to achieve stable perfusion. There are only one or two sites of massive blood loss into the GI tract that are compatible with this clinical scenario. The most usual is the posterior penetrating duodenal ulcer with erosion of the gastroduodenal or inferior pancreaticoduodenal artery. It would be an appropriate step in treatment to continue infusion and transfusion of patient in the operating room, and if the patient remains in shock to open the abdomen and go immediately to the duodenum for control and ligation of the large caliber bleeding vessel if that is what is open in the base of the ulcer. If it is not, aortic compression can help in the resuscitation process while a source of blood loss is estimated by the position of the maximum bleeding rapidly entering the gut. This is sometimes the case at the erosion of a vascular prosthesis into the GI tract, and that might be suggested by any pre-operative history or scar.

In the patient who enters in shock and is briefly resuscitated from it, continuing to actively bleed, a single diagnostic study might be performed, and the highest yield procedure with the safest rapid process toward therapy would be endoscopy.

Endoscopy is useful because it might be helpful in one form of initial therapy if the source of bleeding was from portal hypertension through bleeding esophageal varices. If upper GI endoscopy revealed the source to be duodenal, an emergency operation can then be expeditiously carried out with that ulcer bleeding site targeted. It is important to recognize that the indication for operation is the bleeding, and not the ulcer diathesis. Ulcer disease can be treated medically, or can be treated surgically by a later elective procedure. Vagotomy and gastric resection would be appropriate treatment for the ulcer diathesis, but not for a bleeding duodenal ulcer in a patient who had entered in shock.

The usual bleeding pattern of colonic diverticulosis is that of moderate hemorrhage in which the patient "stutter stops". This bleeding is annoying since it is significant blood loss requiring transfusion up to half or more of the blood volume in 24 hours, but just at the time a diagnostic localization procedure is carried out, the blood flow rate seems to decrease below the sensitivity of the method to find it. Arteriography is useful here since it can not only find the source of bleeding, it may be useful through that catheter to administer pharmacologic therapy to slow visceral flow. Arteriography or endoscopy might be appropriate to localize this flow, but it is unlikely that barium study will be helpful, and should be avoided in the patient with moderate or greater bleeding rates.

For the patient who has occult blood loss the presenting feature is usually anemia and whatever high output cardiac consequences result from it. A barium enema is an appropriate primary diagnostic procedure in this event; arteriography plays a role, and endoscopy may be appropriate, but less for discovery of the bleeding site than for identification of a primary pathology or tumor, which is more likely than a primary ulcer.

Items 214-223

214. Which is the correct statement regarding the vagus nerves?

    (A) they are sympathetic trunks
    (B) the right vagus nerve is anterior on the stomach
    (C) the left vagus nerve is posterior on the stomach
    (D) both vagal trunks send fibers along the lesser curve to the distal stomach
    (E) vagal stimulation inhibits parietal cell acid secretion

215. Which of these therapeutic maneuvers remarkably increases the likelihood of recurrent ulcer?

    (A) high, subtotal gastrectomy
    (B) retained antrum connected to duodenum
    (C) prolonged treatment with ranitidine
    (D) prolonged treatment with omeprazole
    (E) prolonged antacid administration with alkali

216. Duodenal ulcer is a likely event in patients with

    (A) gastrinoma
    (B) gastric carcinoma
    (C) pernicious anemia
    (D) pancreatic cholera (WDHA)
    (E) truncal vagotomy

217. Each of the following are advantages of superselective (parietal cell) vagotomy **EXCEPT**:

    (A) no gastric drainage procedure is necessary
    (B) incidence of diarrhea is reduced
    (C) vagal innervation of biliary tree is not impaired
    (D) no anastomotic suture lines required with risk of leak
    (E) ulcer recurrence rate is abolished

218. Which of these statements is **NOT** true of dumping syndrome?

    (A) it is unlikely with a functioning intact pylorus
    (B) dizziness, palpitations and flushing are common clinical features
    (C) it would be less likely to occur in the prolonged fasting state
    (D) it usually resolves untreated over a short time
    (E) operation is sometimes required to take down the gastric connections to the lower gut

219. Which is the **LEAST** likely cause for upper gastrointestinal bleeding in the patient with known chronic alcoholism?

    (A) gastrinoma
    (B) duodenal ulcer
    (C) gastric mucosal tears (Mallory-Weiss)
    (D) gastroesophageal varices
    (E) erosive gastritis

220. Which of the following studies is most likely to make the diagnosis of a malignant ulcer in gastric carcinoma?

    (A) barium upper GI contrast
    (B) CT scan
    (C) nonhealing on three weeks of treatment
    (D) gastroscopic biopsy
    (E) random nasogastric aspirate for cytology

221. Which of these findings indicates a resection for curative intent in a gastric tumor?

    (A) lower peritoneal mass palpable by rectal exam
    (B) malignant nodule in umbilicus
    (C) gastroscopic biopsy of lymphoma
    (D) malignant ascites
    (E) positive supraclavicular lymph node

222. Which of the following is **NOT** a risk factor for gastric cancer?

    (A) alcoholism
    (B) Oriental race
    (C) blood group O
    (D) pernicious anemia
    (E) smokers

223. Which of the following postoperative supportive measures is **NOT** indicated following total gastrectomy?

    (A) vitamin B-12 replacement
    (B) chloride repletion
    (C) frequent small high calorie feedings
    (D) monitoring of hemoglobin for anemia
    (E) clinical monitoring for metastatic disease

ANSWERS AND TUTORIALS ON ITEMS 214-223

The answers are: **214**-D; **215**-B; **216**-A; **217**-E; **218**-D; **219**-A; **220**-D; **221**-C; **222**-C; **223**-B.

214. The right vagus nerve runs posteriorly and the left vagus nerve anteriorly on the surface of the stomach, but both contribute fibers called "nerves of Latarjet" along the lesser curvature to the distal stomach. The vagus nerve is parasympathetic, and stimulation causes parietal cells to increase acid secretion.

215. Excision of the major portion of the acid secreting stomach reduces the likelihood of ulcer, as do protracted treatments with antacids of alkali, H_2-receptor antagonists, or proton-pump inhibition. However, if antrum is left in contact with duodenum following stomach resection, the physiologic situation called the "Mann-Williamson preparation" exists in which chronic antral gastrin release gives a near inevitability of peptic ulcer recurrence. It is for that reason that many gastric resections are designed for antral exclusion or resection.

216. Patients with pernicious anemia frequently have associated atrophic gastritis with a failure of gastric acid secretion. This is also true for the syndrome known as pancreatic cholera or "watery diarrhea, hypokalemia, and achlorhydria" with which patients also produce less acid. Truncal vagotomy would interrupt the cephalic phase of gastric acid stimulation and gastrectomy would eliminate the acid producing cells, making duodenal ulcer very unlikely.

Patients with gastrinoma (Zollinger-Ellison syndrome) have a sustained autonomous secretion of gastrin which makes peptic ulceration very likely, since whatever parietal cells are present will be under constant stimulation. It is for that reason that total gastrectomy was suggested as a treatment for Zollinger-Ellison syndrome, since if there is "no acid, no ulcer".

217. Selective vagotomy allows other viscera to have intact vagal innervation so that diarrhea incidence is less, and biliary innervation is preserved, although this latter is of questionable significance. Superselective vagotomy denervates only parietal cells in its intent, and therefore motor nerves to the antrum should be spared and no gastric drainage procedure would be necessary. In fact, no entry into the gut is required, and no anastomotic suture lines would be subject to risk.

However, parietal cell vagotomy may require a meticulous procedure that could be incomplete, and this may lead to complications from over-zealous interruption of nerve and vascular supply to the lesser curve and may cause a vascular necrosis of the lesser curvature of the stomach, or less than adequate interruption of all the fibers may lead to recurrence of the ulcer from incomplete denervation.

218. Dumping syndrome occurs when there is a rapid entry of hypertonic gastric contents into the duodenum or jejunum, which is, therefore, very unlikely if the pylorus is present and functioning. If it is bypassed, hypotension may occur from the dilution occasioned by the osmotic load in the gut, and flushing and palpitations are common. Because of the anatomic rerouting of the gastric contents, the syndrome typically does not go away, and is not accommodated within a short period of time from the gastric resection.

Medical therapy is generally successful in ameliorating the condition by decreasing carbohydrates and anticholinergic treatment as well as careful monitoring of fluid intake so as not to drink during meals to allow greater time for gastric mixing. The syndrome does not occur in the fasting state. Only rarely are symptoms so severe and unmanageable that takedown of the gastric bypass is required or a slower mixing of gastric contents engineered by adding resistance to outflow by a reversed antiperistaltic loop of gut.

219. The patient with chronic alcoholism usually has some degree of cirrhosis and portal hypertension. The latter accounts for the likelihood of varices and their propensity to bleed. However, the cirrhosis also decreases histaminase activity in the liver, and all foodstuffs or the blood itself in the gastrointestinal tract will be absorbed and, with its histamines, be absorbed into the portal circulation where the histamine is deaminated in the liver. If the liver is impaired in this process and there is shunting of the histamine to the systemic circulation, the patient is under chronic histamine stimulation for gastric acid production and duodenal ulcer or gastritis may result.

Vomiting is frequently a problem, and the recurrent retching and vomiting may give rise to Mallory-Weiss tears of the gastric lining. Gastrinoma is rare and would have no higher incidence in the alcoholic than is the population at large.

220. Nonhealing of an ulcer on appropriate therapy may be suggestive of malignancy, but is also a property of persistent or recurrent ulcer diathesis. Random gastric fluid sampling for cytologic examination may get lucky with some identification if food particles, blood and other degenerating debris do not confuse sampling, but gastric brushing gives better cytology and gastric biopsy gives the definitive diagnosis. Both barium radiography and CT would only give suggestions as to characteristic shape, but the definitive procedure for differentiation is gastric biopsy.

221. The implants within the peritoneum or at distant sites have been described as contraindications: the supraclavicular lymph node (Virchow's node), the "Blumer's shelf" palpable by rectal exam, or the "Sister Mary Joseph's node" in the umbilicus or malignant ascites detected by paracentesis are all contraindications for curative exploration. In contrast, a diagnosis of lymphoma by gastroscopy is actually a helpful sign, since gastrectomy for lymphoma rather than adenocarcinoma has a much better prognosis following surgical attempt at cure.

222. The highest incidence of gastric cancer is seen in Japan and the Orient, and it is highest in lower socioeconomic groups with a high intake of alcohol and tobacco. Pernicious anemia patients have low acid secretion and are at higher risk. It is blood group A that is associated with a higher incidence, and other evidence of genetic linkage is two to six times the risk in a positive family history.

223. One of the principle problems following gastrectomy is maintenance of a normal hemoglobin, since vitamin B-12 absorption is made possible by intrinsic factor and can be replaced with vitamin B-12 administration. It is frequently difficult to maintain weight in the absence of the stomach, since the capacitance for food intake is reduced, and dumping or diarrhea may follow as well. Frequent feeding and a check on the caloric intake is important nutritional follow-up, and there should be monitoring to differentiate the weight loss and cachexia of metastatic recurrent disease from that of nutritional crippling from the absence of the stomach. There is no need to replace chloride, since it is not being secreted by the stomach, and in any event when secreted when the stomach is present, it is reabsorbed, so there is no net loss of this abundant anion in the changes following gastrectomy.

Items 224-233

224. Which is the **LEAST** likely cause of duodenal obstruction that might be expected to be encountered in the patient with gastric outlet obstruction?

    (A) primary duodenal carcinoma
    (B) pancreatic carcinoma
    (C) duodenal stenosis from healed ulcer
    (D) benign polyp or leiomyoma
    (E) benign or malignant biliary pathology encroaching on the duodenum

225. Duodenal obstruction in the newborn is **LEAST** likely to be associated with which of the following?

    (A) pyloric stenosis
    (B) duodenal web
    (C) annular pancreas
    (D) bowel malrotation
    (E) ulceration and stenosis

226. Which of the following characteristics of an anterior perforating duodenal ulcer is **LEAST** likely?

    (A) exsanguinating hemorrhage
    (B) rigid board-like abdomen
    (C) abrupt onset in a previously well unsuspecting patient
    (D) normal amylase
    (E) an acute abdominal emergency

227. A 32 year-old patient with known duodenal ulcer under treatment becomes pale, sweaty and faint. His abdominal X-ray shows no free air, but he has epigastric tenderness and an amylase of 850 mg/dl. The most likely urgent crisis he faces is

   (A) fulminant pancreatitis
   (B) peritoneal soilage and peritonitis
   (C) life-threatening hemorrhage
   (D) pancreatic pseudocyst
   (E) gastric outlet obstruction

228. Afferent loop syndrome is **LEAST** likely to result in which of the following complications?

   (A) recurrent ulcer
   (B) duodenal stump blowout
   (C) bacterial overgrowth
   (D) bloating from distention and necrosis
   (E) carcinogenesis

229. Which of the following neoplasms is **MOST** frequently sited in the duodenum?

   (A) primary adenocarcinoma
   (B) gastrinoma
   (C) metastatic colonic adenocarcinoma
   (D) lymphoma
   (E) leiomyosarcoma

230. Duodenal mucosa does **NOT** secrete which of the following?

   (A) hydrochloric acid
   (B) gastrin
   (C) secretin
   (D) cholecystokinin
   (E) enterogastrone

231. In a gastroduodenostomy (Billroth I) complications may result, including all of the following **EXCEPT**:

   (A) afferent loop syndrome
   (B) alkaline reflux gastritis
   (C) duodenal ulcer recurrence
   (D) dumping
   (E) gastric stasis

232. Which of the following stimulations to gastric acid secretion is **NOT** mediated by histamine and cannot be blocked by H_2-receptor antagonists?

   (A)   cephalic phase
   (B)   gastric phase
   (C)   duodenal G cells
   (D)   gastrin from pancreatic islet cells
   (E)   intestinal phase

233. Which of the following agents does **NOT** break down the mucosal barrier to back-diffusion of H^+?

   (A)   alcohol
   (B)   prostaglandin
   (C)   salicylates
   (D)   bile salts
   (E)   potassium concentration

ANSWERS AND TUTORIALS ON ITEMS 224-233

The answers are: **224-A; 225-E; 226-A; 227-C; 228-E; 229-B; 230-A; 231-A; 232-E; 233-B**.

224. The malignant potential obstruction in the duodenum is that of surrounding organ primary disease, since malignancy in the duodenum is the lowest in frequency of any primary site along the gastrointestinal tract. Benign strictures of the duodenum may take place from inflammation and recurrent fibrotic healing with stenosis that results, most frequently from duodenal ulcer, but may be from biliary or pancreatic origin as well. The most frequent carcinomas that give rise to gastric outlet obstruction, are those that originate in the pancreas.

225. The congenital causes of duodenal obstruction are anatomic abnormalities that are first noted after birth such as duodenal web, atresia, or annular pancreas, or the anatomic derangement from a failure of fusion fascia that normally situate the abdominal viscera that results in malrotation and "Ladd's bands". Pyloric stenosis is acquired later in life of the infant when it is detected a month or more after birth, but duodenal ulceration would be very unlikely, and chronicity of such an ulcer to the point of fibrotic stenosis would be unheard of, making ulcerative stenosis the least likely cause of gastric outlet obstruction of the newborn.

226. Posterior penetrating duodenal ulcers bleed. Anterior duodenal ulcers perforate. The latter give a previously well patient an abrupt catastrophic intra-abdominal emergency with peritonitis as gastric contents flood the peritoneum and a board-like rigid abdomen results. The posterior penetrating ulcer is usually a more chronic phenomenon in which the ulceration is known or suspected previously, and erodes back into the pancreas giving pancreatitis and the erosive enzymatic digestion of very large visceral blood vessels that can cause exsanguination.

227. The posterior penetrating ulcer has reached this patient's pancreas causing the pancreatitis and the elevated amylase. Both fulminant pancreatitis and its much later sequel of pancreatic pseudocyst are manageable in most instances, as would be gastric outlet obstruction. It is unlikely that he will perforate, since the posterior location of the ulcer makes communication with the free peritoneum unlikely with a lesser risk of peritonitis.

The biggest threat to life in this individual is the proximity of the major blood supply in this area, the gastroduodenal and the pancreaticoduodenal arteries which lie in the inflammatory mass of autodigestive enzymes and gastric acid output. The hemorrhage that results from disruption of these vessels is catastrophic, and requires treatment — even in advance of precise diagnosis — and such a patient is taken to the operating room, not for radiographic or endoscopic confirmation, since abrupt loss of half or more of the blood volume over a short period of time is not coming from mucosal origin alone. Life-threatening hemorrhage is the risk associated with posterior penetration of duodenal ulcer.

228. The afferent loop in a Billroth-II reconstruction following partial gastrectomy may become obstructed at the gastrojejunal stoma, and the afferent loop may become distended. This distention can give stasis with bacterial overgrowth.

The duodenal stump may blow out if pressure buildup occurs and recurrent ulceration and necrosis are possible. Although each of these significant complications is part of the afferent loop syndrome, none are implicated in malignant degeneration, and the long-term risk of cancer in the afferent loop syndrome is not a problem.

229. The duodenum is a site remarkable in the GI tract for its low incidence of adenocarcinoma. However, there are other secretory cells in the mucosa, and some of these are endocrine. These endocrine cells may become the site of excessive gastrin secretion. As many as 10% or more of patients with Zollinger-Ellison syndrome may have a duodenal gastrinoma. Lymphoma is possible in the duodenum but not at a higher rate than anywhere along the gastrointestinal tract, and adenocarcinoma from the colon is rarely metastatic in this site preferring travel along lymphatics in the mesentery. Leiomyosarcoma is possible wherever smooth muscle is present, but is very rare in general, and exceedingly so in the duodenum.

230. The enteroendocrine cells located within the duodenum can produce many peptides and do so in physiologic response to duodenal filling when secretin, gastrin, and cholecystokinin are released and enterogastrone inhibits rapid emptying of the stomach. The mucosal goblet cells produce exocrine secretions of mucus, but there are no parietal cells that secrete hydrochloric acid. There may be ectopic "rests" along the gastrointestinal tract at embryologic sites such as the Meckel's diverticulum that contain gastric mucosa and can secrete hydrochloric acid, but these are not typically found in the duodenum. The duodenum is sensitive to hydrochloric acid in high concentrations, and for that reason direct anastomosis with gastric acid secreting cells without the pylorus in between or without modification of the parietal cell secretion of hydrochloric acid is injurious to the duodenum and may give rise to recurrent ulceration.

231. The Billroth I gastroduodenostomy directly connects the stump of the stomach to the duodenum, end-to-end in most instances, without an afferent loop as exists with Billroth II gastrojejunostomy. Because the pylorus is destroyed, dumping is possible, and because the anastomosis may be in the area that has been inflamed previously or might become so with recurrent ulcer disease possible, stenosis and gastric stasis may result in some instances. Because the biliary input now has retrograde access into the stomach, alkaline reflux gastritis is possible. Of the complications listed, the only one not possible is the afferent loop syndrome since there is no afferent loop in gastroduodenostomy.

232. The cephalic phase of gastric acid stimulation is by vagal efferents which stimulate parietal cells and the G cells through histamine release. That same effect comes from gastrin whether from gastric, duodenal, or pancreatic islet origin, each of which have a histamine intermediary and therefore are capable of being blocked by an antihistamine that is antagonistic to H_2 receptors. The intestinal phase has another group of enteric endocrine peptides, not all of which are histamine intermediated, and therefore are not uniformly susceptible to interception with an H_2-receptor antagonist.

233. The mucosal barrier is sensitive to the H^+ secreted in highly concentrated form by the gastric parietal cells. That duodenal mucosa is further sensitive to the H^+ in the presence of alcohol, salicylate, and bile salts, and concentrated potassium may cause erosion as well. Prostaglandin has been used experimentally to improve the mucosal barrier and protect it from ulceration, and is a suggested future treatment for the peptic ulcer diathesis.

Items 234-243

234. The most common cancer in the liver is

    (A)   hepatoma
    (B)   cholangiocarcinoma
    (C)   hepatocholangioma
    (D)   fibrolamellar
    (E)   metastatic

235. The anatomic division of the liver for right lobar hepatectomy may be defined by each of the following **EXCEPT**:

    (A)   the falciform ligament
    (B)   the distribution of the right hepatic artery
    (C)   the distribution of the right portal vein
    (D)   the drainage area of the right hepatic veins
    (E)   an imaginary line drawn through the gallbladder fossa to the vena cava

236. Alpha-fetoprotein is **NOT** useful and **NOT** indicated for

    (A) primary screening for hepatoma
    (B) detection of persistent tumor after resection
    (C) detection of recurrence during follow-up after therapy
    (D) an indication for adjunctive chemotherapy
    (E) help in indicating reoperation or thrombosis of tumor

237. One method of pre-operative therapy that has been helpful in facilitating liver resection for tumor has been

    (A) pre-operative external beam radiation
    (B) arteriographic vascular occlusion
    (C) portal venous thrombosis
    (D) intensive cancer chemotherapy with leucovorin rescue
    (E) three weeks of total parenteral nutrition

238. If the residual, well-vascularized, hepatic remnant is normal and not involved with cirrhotic fibrosis or inflammation, what is the maximum portion of functioning liver that can be removed with normal survival?

    (A) 10%
    (B) 25%
    (C) 40%
    (D) 60%
    (E) 80%

239. Of the following transmissible agents that may give rise to focal liver infections, which may cause an anaphylactic response if the contents are spilled in the event of resection or rupture?

    (A) *Entamoeba histolytica*
    (B) *Staphylococcus aureus*
    (C) *Clonorchis sinensis*
    (D) *Echinococcus granulosus*
    (E) *Proteus mirabilis*

240. A 24 year-old woman experiences an acute abdomen with hemorrhage and shock following minor trauma when falling over a chair and striking her abdomen. At operation, a ruptured tumor in the liver is encountered. The only medicine she has ever taken has been oral contraceptives for the past seven years. The likely diagnosis is

   (A) hepatoma
   (B) arteriovenous malformation
   (C) fibronodular hyperplasia
   (D) endometrioma
   (E) metastatic adenocarcinoma

241. Which of the following statements is **NOT** true concerning pylephlebitis?

   (A) it is caused by bacteria in the urinary collecting system
   (B) it may lead to portal vein thrombosis
   (C) it is frequently associated with hepatic abscess
   (D) patients typically have severe illness in sepsis
   (E) the bacterial origin is often from the colon

242. Which statement about cancer in the liver is true?

   (A) primary hepatoma and metastatic liver cancer each exhibit 85% or better 5-year survival
   (B) primary hepatoma has an 85% 5-year survival but metastatic liver cancer shows less than 10% 5-year survival
   (C) primary hepatoma shows less than 10% 5-year survival but metastatic liver cancer shows greater than 80% 5-year survival
   (D) both primary hepatoma and metastatic liver cancer show equivalent survivals with equivalent average duration of survival
   (E) primary hepatoma and metastatic liver cancer each show less than 10% 5-year survival

243. Each of the following factors are important in determining operability and resectability of a liver tumor **EXCEPT**:

   (A) the patient's age
   (B) number of liver segments involved in tumor and resection proposed
   (C) prothrombin time
   (D) presence or absence of cirrhosis in the residual liver following proposed resection
   (E) ongoing active hepatitis

ANSWERS AND TUTORIALS ON ITEMS 234-243

The answers are: **234-E; 235-A; 236-A; 237-B; 238-E; 239-D; 240-C; 241-A; 242-E; 243-C**.

234. In the US, hepatoma is much less common than other primary adenocarcinomas in the GI tract, particularly of the colon. Any tumor that disseminates by way of the portal circulation from the gut has a propensity for hepatic metastases, which are the vast majority of cancers in the liver that originate elsewhere in the gut.

235. The anatomic division of the liver is very important for the three part blood flow which is an important consideration in hepatic resection. The neat anatomic division of the falciform ligament actually separates the left lateral lobe of the liver from the median superior and median inferior components of the left lobe and it is not the true dividing line for hepatic lobectomy. The right and left lobes are divided through an anatomic line that would pass through the gallbladder fossa to the vena cava, which correlates with the distribution of the right hepatic artery, portal and venous systems.

236. Alpha-fetoprotein is helpful after the diagnosis of hepatoma in following the patient through treatment, but has not been useful or cost-effective for screening for primary diagnosis and is not so indicated. It may be helpful to serve as a proxy for the presence of the tumor when the level had previously fallen after treatment and the elevations in alpha-fetoprotein secondarily may indicate treatment without further collateral proof of recurrence.

237. Hepatoma is not a radiosensitive tumor and no pre-operative utility would be expected from radiotherapy or intensive cytotoxic chemotherapy, since it is also highly unresponsive to drug therapy. Immunotherapy and nutritional therapy might make a marginal difference in the host response to operation, but are inadequate to make any marginal difference that would be worth a delay.

The one technique listed that has been proven effective in selective instances is devascularization of the liver segment anticipated to be resected, which gives a head-start on the regeneration of liver function in adjacent liver to be preserved. It is also suggested to decrease the tumor neovascularity involved in the tumor-bearing segment, but this is difficult to judge prospectively and impossible to control in comparative trials. Radiographic occlusion is nonetheless advocated for some selected pre-operative hepatoma management.

238. The liver has amazing abilities of restoration through hyperplasia that allow regeneration of both anatomic mass and physiologic function back to normal following removal of up to 80% of the liver. Not only is this regenerative capacity amazing, but it also seems to know when to stop! The factors which govern this regenerative capacity have been studied and remain an intriguing puzzle, but messenger RNA is involved.

239. Pyogenic abscesses, such as that with *Staphylococcus* or *Proteus* may cause febrile reactions and can lead to septicemia, but not hypersensitivity reactions. *Clonorchis sinensis* is an

Oriental liver fluke that takes up residence in the biliary tree, and is a source of inflammatory response, but not anaphylaxis. Amoeba are protozoans that in some zymogen classes not only give rise to colonic inflammation but invade the portal blood stream and can set up hepatic abscess, which when drained does not give anaphylaxis. This is not the case with hydatid cyst caused by *Echinococcus granulosus*. Not only can rupture of the cyst result in implantation and dissemination of daughter cysts, *Echinococcus* can cause a lethal hypersensitivity reaction as well if spilled into the peritoneum.

240. Hepatic nodular hyperplasia is the so-called "pill tumor" found in young women who have had prolonged exposure to oral contraceptive agents with progestational combinations. A young patient is unlikely to have either primary hepatoma or metastatic carcinoma in the liver at her age with no antecedent history of ill health or medication, and arteriovenous malformations don't often rupture into the abdominal cavity. An endometrioma is a possibility, but unlikely to produce hemorrhage in its superficial implantation of the severity that would give shock. The "pill tumor" often presents with hemorrhage following minimal abdominal trauma and this incidental discovery is often the only way this otherwise benign lesion is recognized — as it became known when first described.

241. Pyelonephritis is not to be confused with pylephlebitis which is an inflammation of the portal vein, most often because of bacterial infection. This bacterial infection frequently originates in the colon, and this blood-borne bacterial infection causes inflammation within the portal system and is often associated with hepatic abscesses with the patient severely ill in sepsis. The urinary tract is not drained by the portal system, and there should be no connection of these anatomic regions despite the confusion in similar sounding names between pylephlebitis and pyelonephritis.

242. There is a mean period of average survival for primary hepatoma that is about three times greater than that for metastatic liver cancer, but neither show a favorable prognosis despite treatment. Few survivors of either diagnosis are alive one year from diagnosis.

243. Each of the factors determine whether sufficient viable liver can be expected to remain to support life in the patient in the event that resection must encompass three segments or greater than 85% of the liver parenchyma, or whether the section of liver remaining is necrotic, cirrhotic or inflamed with hepatitis. There is a greater capacity for regeneration in the younger patient, and advanced age would rule out 80% hepatectomy for the compromised reserves that would need to be called upon. Prothrombin time is a measure of the liver production of a labile clotting factor, that can be reconstituted with vitamin K administration that would correct the prothrombin time even if it were prolonged.

Items 244-253

244. Each of the following conditions exhibits splenomegaly **EXCEPT**:

    (A) early acute malaria
    (B) Gaucher's disease
    (C) myelofibrosis
    (D) end-stage chronic malaria
    (E) hypersplenism

245. Splenic repair rather that splenectomy should be attempted in all of the following conditions **EXCEPT**:

    (A) multiple trauma with severe head injury and extremity fractures
    (B) stab wound to the spleen
    (C) avulsion of splenic capsule from short gastric arteries during vagotomy
    (D) splenic vein tear during pancreatic exploration
    (E) 8 year-old boy with arm fracture, abdominal bruise following a fall from tree with positive abdominal tap and normal blood pressure

246. Each of the following conditions is an indication for splenectomy **EXCEPT**:

    (A) thrombocytopenia
    (B) traumatic splenic laceration in a child with minimum blood loss
    (C) a splenic artery aneurysm within the splenic pulp
    (D) splenic abscess
    (E) hereditary spherocytosis

247. Surgical identification and excision of an accessory spleen is important in

    (A) splenectomy for hematologic indication
    (B) staging laparotomy
    (C) splenectomy for trauma
    (D) splenosis
    (E) factor VIII deficiency

248. Adjunctive methods that may facilitate splenectomy for hematologic disease and benefit the patient include each of the following **EXCEPT**:

    (A) polyvalent pneumococcal vaccine
    (B) heparinization
    (C) platelet transfusion
    (D) corticosteroids
    (E) immediate splenic artery ligation

249. Each of the following results after splenectomy would be considered complications because they are not part of the normal expected post-splenectomy course **EXCEPT**:

    (A) pancreatitis
    (B) thrombocytosis
    (C) subphrenic abscess
    (D) hemorrhage requiring reoperation
    (E) anemia

250. Which of the following conditions is expected to co-exist with hypersplenism in a patient with hereditary spherocytosis?

    (A) thrombophlebitis
    (B) gallstones
    (C) bone pain
    (D) repeated crises of general abdominal pain
    (E) extramedullary myelopoiesis

251. Each of the organisms listed may be associated with severe septicemia eight years following splenectomy in a 4 year-old child **EXCEPT**:

    (A) *Pneumococcus*
    (B) *Pseudomonas*
    (C) *Hemophilus*
    (D) *Neisseria*
    (E) *Meningococcus*

252. One factor weighing **AGAINST** splenectomy in a patient with splenomegaly from myelofibrosis is

    (A) a potential for painful splenic infarction
    (B) the threat of intra-abdominal hemorrhage
    (C) the majority of blood forming cells may be in the spleen
    (D) displacement of abdominal viscera by the massive splenic enlargement
    (E) the operative risk of the splenectomy for massive splenomegaly

253. Splenectomy for hereditary spherocytosis is curative for which of the following abnormalities?

    (A) anemia
    (B) osmotic red cell fragility
    (C) cholecystitis
    (D) iron absorption
    (E) spherocytosis

ANSWERS AND TUTORIALS ON ITEMS 244-253

The answers are: **244-D; 245-A; 246-B; 247-A; 248-B; 249-B; 250-B; 251-B; 252-C; 253-A**.

244. The early stages of malaria have splenomegaly as a prominent feature, particularly in children. In fact, an epidemiologic survey method for determining the prevalence of malaria is the splenomegaly rate in the pediatric population. Over repeated attacks, the spleen suffers multiple sequential infarcts and eventually fibroses down to the small fibrotic organ that is not only clinically not palpable, but in some instances not discoverable on surgical exploration following this "autosplenectomy".

Gaucher's disease is a glucocerebroside accumulation disorder due to deficiency in lysosomal glucocerebrosidase which produces some of the largest spleens recorded. Myelofibrosis, from its extramedullary myeloproliferative disorders, also produces massive splenomegaly in nearly all cases, and hypersplenism is the product of a spleen that is much enlarged as a rule. Of the options listed, only end-stage malaria exhibits a spleen that is not only not palpable clinically, but most likely shriveled below normal size which approximates about 150 grams in the average adult.

245. Splenic conservation should be attempted whenever it is safe and appropriate, particularly in the young. That would include both trauma as described for the boy who fell from a tree or a knife stab wound as well. It particularly applies to intra-operative incidental injuries such as that encountered during vagotomy or pancreatic exploration. However, it has no place in the patient with severe multiple injuries, when the time and attention devoted to splenic repair would pose excessive risk in view of multiple systems which require operative attention.

246. Thrombocytopenia from idiopathic or other acquired origins may respond to splenectomy if steroid therapy no longer induces a response in raising platelets. Spherocytosis is a frequent hemolytic indication for splenectomy as one of the only treatments and with excellent success rate. Splenic abscess and splenic artery aneurysm both are treated by splenectomy if simple drainage is inadequate or an exterior splenic artery aneurysmectomy is not possible. In children, however, splenectomy is to be avoided for trauma unless there is hemodynamic instability and no other way to control the intra-abdominal hemorrhage. With minimal blood loss and stable vital signs, minimal splenic disruption can be managed by observation in order that the splenic filtration and immunologic function be preserved. If surgical exploration is undertaken, attempts at repair of minor traumatic splenic injuries are recommended, particularly in children, and splenectomy reserved for unsalvageable disruption or patients with multiple other injuries requiring urgent attention.

247. To control consumption of blood cells and platelets, all accessible splenic tissue should be excised, including that in ectopic or accessory locations. Such exploration and excision is not indicated in staging laparotomy, and no disturbance of any splenic tissue not actively bleeding or irreparable should be attempted for trauma. Splenosis is the implantation of viable splenic fragments, and would be irrelevant except if there were hematologic abnormalities secondary to these fragments. At one time, factor VIII deficiency was thought to be improved with splenic implant, and although disproved, there would be no indication for removal of splenic tissue.

248. In dealing with splenomegaly, particularly of the hyperactive spleen which is engorged with blood and consuming platelets and other blood cells, early splenic artery ligation as soon as exposure permits is important, while venous "autotransfusion" from the enlarged spleen continues as the spleen is mobilized. At this point, the patient would be able to retain transfused platelets, which would help in hemostasis for the operative dissection. Prior vaccination of pneumococcal vaccine would protect to some degree from at least some strains of encapsulated gram-positive organisms for which splenectomized patients are at risk.

Heparin anticoagulation would be contraindicated, and would make hemostasis more difficult in the patient already likely to bleed, particularly in the large potential space left behind following excision of an enlarged spleen.

249. The potential space left behind may fill with some minimal bleeding, but reoperation for hemorrhage control is a complication. Subphrenic abscess is not unheard of, but should be brought to a near-zero level by meticulous attention to technique and represents a significant complication when it occurs. The same attention to technique will avoid injury to the tail of the pancreas which lies in close proximity to the splenic hilum, since distal pancreatic injury may give rise to some degree of pancreatitis which is dangerous considering the ligated vessels and the enzymatic sequelae of pancreatic injury, particularly with a patient with impaired clotting abilities. Anemia signifies inadequate blood replacement or a continuing blood loss, and the postoperative red cell indices should be normal.

Thrombocytosis is a normal and expected result of complete splenic ablation. The platelet count should rise to levels that are expected to be approximately two to five times normal for a period of up to a year, but would require no treatment unless the platelet count of more than $10^6/mm^3$ persists.

250. The breakdown products of splenic filtration of spherocytes include the heavy pigment load to the liver for excretion, with pigmented gallstones being so likely as to recommend cholecystectomy for patients undergoing splenectomy for this indication. Sequential repeated abdominal pain crises and bone pain are characteristic of sickle cell anemia from ischemic attacks and infarcts when hypoxic. Thrombophlebitis is no more common in patients with red cell disorders than in the general population, and in a patient with hypersplenism the thrombosis would be less likely. Although the production of replacements for the red cells removed from circulation would be speeded up, in this condition the bone marrow has sufficient reserves that extramedullary sources are not likely to be involved.

251. Gram-positive encapsulated organisms are most typically associated with severe sepsis following splenectomy, and *Pneumococcus* is the principle species. *Hemophilus*, *Meningococcus* and *Neisseria* share the capsular characteristics of the organisms responsible for post-splenectomy sepsis syndrome, but *Pseudomonas* does not.

252. An operative risk is always a consideration, but splenectomy is not a very technically demanding operation even when the spleen is massively enlarged. In fact, mobilization of the massive spleen is sometimes easier, since it becomes a midline abdominal organ with very large and quite easily identifiable and relatively constant vascular attachments. Splenic infarction and the pain and risk of hemorrhage associated with it is a serious consideration indicating splenectomy as is the discomfort from the enlarged spleen moving around the abdomen and displacing other abdominal viscera or causing early satiety following meals.

A very real risk of splenectomy in a patient with myelofibrosis is that the majority of hematopoietic cells are in the enlarged spleen, and the patient may have an impaired ability to produce blood cells requiring transfusion for an extended period if there exists a "packed marrow" that no longer has capacity to produce blood.

253. Splenectomy should reduce hemolysis and therefore correct anemia long-term. The operation would have no effect on iron absorption, nor the continued production of red cells that exhibit osmotic fragility and spherocytic morphology. The excessive pigment breakdown load delivered to the liver for excretion even early in life had most likely produced pigmented gallstones; and, this occurrence, which is present even in children, is not reversed by splenectomy.

Items 254-263

254. Adenocarcinoma of the colon is

 (A) more common than skin cancer
 (B) significantly higher in men than women in the US
 (C) geographically distributed across the globe
 (D) the most frequent visceral cancer in the US
 (E) often cured by chemotherapy

255. Which of the following conditions is **NOT** a risk factor in predilection for the development of colon cancer?

 (A) gender
 (B) genetics
 (C) diet
 (D) age
 (E) environment

256. Which of these antecedent conditions predisposes to the higher risk of the development of colon cancer?

    (A) Crohn's disease
    (B) ulcerative colitis
    (C) diverticulosis
    (D) urinary bladder cancer
    (E) melanoma

257. The principle population screening method for detecting colo-rectal abnormalities is

    (A) barium enema
    (B) sigmoidoscopy
    (C) digital rectal exam
    (D) occult fecal blood
    (E) colonoscopy

258. The most likely cause of occult blood loss in a 68 year-old who undergoes routine physical examination after retirement is

    (A) hemorrhoids
    (B) *fissure-in-ano*
    (C) diverticulosis
    (D) carcinoma
    (E) adenomatous polyp

259. An annular "napkin ring" appearance on barium enema is most characteristic of

    (A) carcinoma of the cecum
    (B) squamous epidermoid cancer of the anus
    (C) cancer of the sigmoid colon
    (D) cancer of the rectal ampulla
    (E) villous adenoma

260. The highest percentage of colon cancers are first found in the

    (A) liver
    (B) cecum
    (C) ascending colon
    (D) descending colon
    (E) rectosigmoid

261. The design of curative operations for colon cancer resections are patterned according to

    (A) the ease of operative excision
    (B) the instruments available for surgical utilization
    (C) the anatomic distribution of adjacent lymphatics
    (D) the minimum colon required for fluid reabsorption
    (E) siting of colostomy

262. Indications for colon resection in a patient with a large sigmoid carcinoma and hepatic metastases include each of the following **EXCEPT**:

    (A) relief of bowel obstruction
    (B) the best chance for a cure
    (C) control of hemorrhage
    (D) prevention of necrosis
    (E) disobstruction of the ureter

263. Which of the following studies is contraindicated in defining the extent of a partial obstruction?

    (A) colonoscopy
    (B) gastrograffin swallow
    (C) barium enema
    (D) barium UGI
    (E) gastrograffin enema

ANSWERS AND TUTORIALS ON ITEMS 254-263

The answers are: **254-D; 255-A; 256-B; 257-D; 258-D; 259-C; 260-E; 261-C; 262-B; 263-D**.

254. The incidence of colon cancer is second only to skin cancers, in the US, but a majority of the skin cancers are trivial with respect to threat to life. Adenocarcinoma of the colon is the most frequent visceral cancer in the US constituting 14% of all nonskin cancers in both males and females which it affects equally. There is a remarkable asymmetry in geographic distribution, since it is nearly unknown in less developed parts of the world and is a component part of Western life style and diseases of development. It is very much a surgical disease, since chemotherapy offers very little palliation and no curative control.

255. Colon cancer constitutes 14% of visceral cancers in males and an identical percentage in females. That there may be a greater number of females at advanced age than males means that the prevalence of colon cancer is higher in females only because of this longevity and not because of a predilection based in biology or behavior difference between the sexes.

An increasing incidence of colon cancer is correlated strongly with an increase in age, and genetic predisposition appears evident from two to three times greater incidence in family members of those affected. However, this is difficult to separate from the environmental factors which are overwhelmingly obvious, since people from areas of the world where colon cancer is nearly unheard of can immigrate to Western urban centers and adopt the life style of modernization and within a generation develop an incidence of colon cancer that sometimes surpasses that of the indigenous Westerners. Some part of this environment is provably associated with low fiber, high fat and refined carbohydrate.

256. There appears to be a random association of colon cancer with other coincident tumors such as melanoma or urinary bladder cancer, but there is a correlation with breast carcinoma and a strong association with carcinoid. Inflammatory disease of the bowel is sharply distinguished between Crohn's disease, which does not appear to be a predisposing risk factor, and ulcerative colitis which has a very high correlation with later development of adenocarcinoma of the colon increasing with duration of the colitis. The anatomic finding of diverticulosis may be associated with same proximate causes — for example, low fiber diet and Western life style, but there is no correlation of the diverticulosis and colon cancer risk primarily.

257. Since the principle easily detected physical finding associated with colon carcinoma is occult blood loss in the stool, this method is a sensitive way of case finding. However, it is very non-specific. For that reason, the much more specific studies of radiographic barium, or physical examination by rectal exam, sigmoidoscopy, or colonoscopy are indicated for those of the general population who screen positive on the more sensitive examination which will uncover a large number of patients who are false positives or who have benign problems discovered by true positive occult blood detection.

258. Hemorrhoids are common, but bleeding from them less so, which is more common with *fissure-in-ano*. However, both of these do not produce occult blood loss but streaking that is visible to the patient. Diverticulosis can cause blood loss, but it is typically not occult when it happens, as it does infrequently, when it may cause massive bleeding. An adenomatous polyp rarely bleeds unless it is large enough to be ischemic, and then often blood loss is part of its passage. The important point to be carried from this question to the clinic is that colon cancer is the single most common cause of occult blood loss in the older patient.

259. Adenocarcinoma of the colon grows into the bowel wall and spreads along the submucosal lymphatics, which are arranged in a circumferential pattern in an area where the structure and function of the colon is principally for propulsion. In the right side of the colon the principle functions are capacitance and water absorption, and tumors tend toward endophytic polypoid growth — although there is frequent overlap between these patterns. Villous adenoma is a frond-like extension that may be sessile when seen on barium enema, but is characteristically polypoid rather than annular wherever it occurs.

Although not principally annular in configuration, both rectal ampulla and perineal lesions would not be described as napkin rings on barium enema, since barium enema does not define the pattern in the lower reaches of the rectum and anus since the barium does not opacify them and there is a rectal ballooned catheter present that interferes with definition on radiographs of this lower extreme end of the colon.

260. The rule of thumb — if not of index finger — is that one-third of colon carcinomas are found within range of digital rectal exam and two-thirds within the range of the sigmoidoscope, or 25 cm. Less frequent are the cancers on the right side of the colon, but they often — but not always — are associated with characteristic clinical syndromes. The majority of colon cancers still offer presentation from symptoms relating to the colon, rather than to metastatic sites such as the liver.

261. Curative resection of colon cancers encompasses not only the area of the primary tumor and adjacent bowel, but also the mesenteric fan or lymphatic distribution in encompassing not only the primary tumor but the most likely sites of potential metastatic spread *en bloc*. These lymphatics closely follow the pattern of portal venous effluent, so the extension is often carried back to the root of the major venous drainage of this region of the bowel. Ease of operation, the instrumentation available, and siting of the stoma are technical considerations as well as the residual colon and its storage and reabsorption capacity for the patient, but each is secondary to the primary concern that the patient undergo a curative resection procedure.

262. Palliative operations for sigmoid cancer are limited in indication if the patient does not have morbidity directly related to the presence of the tumor. These factors would include continuing blood loss or necrosing tumor with the threat of bowel disruption. Bowel obstruction should certainly be relieved, but it is not generally a good idea to perform this much in advance of imminent obstruction, since the patient's survival may be a shorter time than the obstruction requires to develop, and this interval would best be served for the patient's own uses rather than hospitalization and recovery. Ureteral obstruction is rare, and typically does not impair renal function if the opposite kidney is uninvolved, but may cause pain and may be relieved incidentally during operation for other indication. A patient is not curable with hepatic metastases already present, and therefore the operation should be limited in scope, without effort to encompass all secondary metastatic areas of spread, since tertiary levels are already involved. The design of the operation will be tailored for the strategy of the indication, namely symptomatic palliation.

263. High grade obstruction in the GI tract, particularly in such an area as the left colon where it may frequently occur, may be studied safely from below with barium or gastrograffin contrast and colonoscopy, since such introduced materials are retrievable. Barium introduced by mouth must be able to pass through the gastrointestinal tract, however, and in the event of a partial high grade bowel obstruction, the oral barium contrast can complete the obstruction making it difficult to retrieve not only the barium, but to pass anything else through the gut and require emergency operation. Judicious use of gastrograffin contrast, conscious of its osmotic activity, can be employed in these instances, but the proximal part of the bowel is already likely to be distended upstream from a site of obstruction, and such bowel distention can decompensate with additional osmotic intraluminal pressure increase. A general rule for partial bowel obstruction is that such obstructions should be studied from the downstream side, that is, distal from the point of obstruction.

CHAPTER III
CARDIOVASCULAR AND THORACIC SURGERY

Items 264-266

A 60 year-old patient had a "coin lesion" in the right apex on chest X-ray. PPD skin test was positive, and bronchial washings were negative. Following antimicrobial therapy, right upper lobectomy was carried out and the cut specimen is shown in **Figure 3.1**.

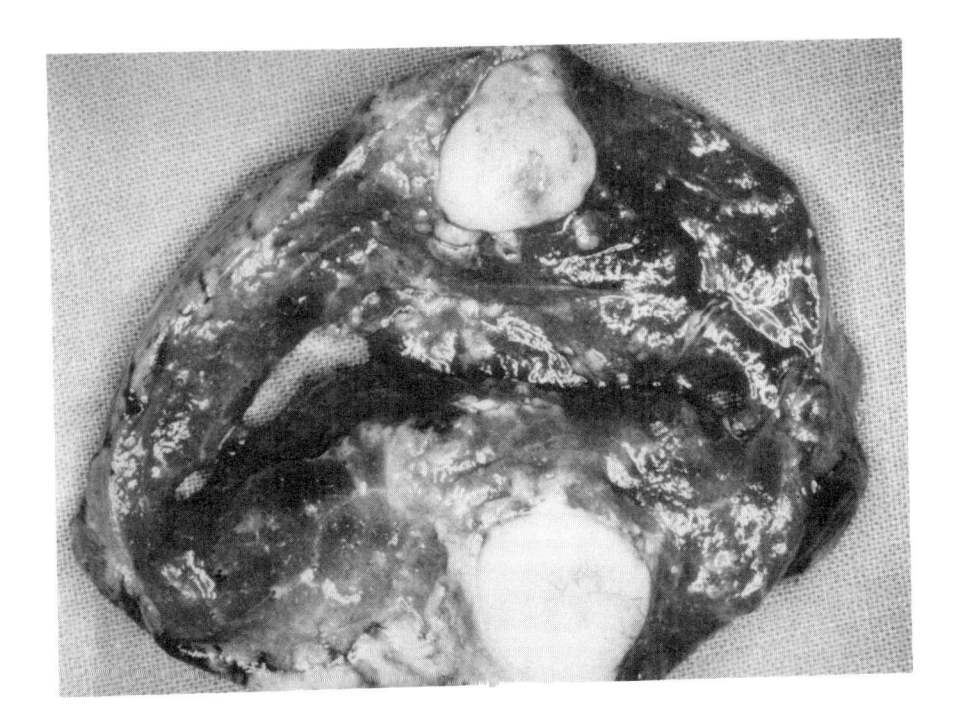

Figure 3.1

264. The specimen shows what is likely a

    (A)   hamartoma of the lung
    (B)   tuberculous granuloma
    (C)   adenocarcinoma
    (D)   "scar carcinoma" of the lung
    (E)   epidermoid carcinoma

265. Operation was carried out to

    (A) keep this lesion from spreading
    (B) rule out malignancy
    (C) prevent later carcinogenesis
    (D) facilitate antimicrobial therapy
    (E) prevent cavitation

266. The differential diagnosis of solitary coin lesions includes each of the following **EXCEPT**:

    (A) carcinoma of the lung
    (B) metastatic adenocarcinoma
    (C) fungal infection
    (D) sarcoid
    (E) hamartoma

ANSWERS AND TUTORIAL ON ITEMS 264-266

The answers are: **264-B; 265-B; 266-D**.

This patient has a tuberculous granuloma, located in its usual position in the lung. The operation was to rule out malignancy in a coin lesion. Since the diagnosis of a coin lesion has a differential that includes carcinoma of the lung in that which will most likely be treated by operation, the differential also considered is that of the other options listed with the exception of sarcoid. Sarcoid does not give a coin lesion but is largely a butterfly pattern along the hilum of lymphatic involvement.

Items 267-269

A patient with end-stage renal failure supported by dialysis developed increasing congestive heart failure and chest pain. The patient died before thoracotomy could be carried out, and the heart is shown in **Figure 3.2** after the pericardium is opened.

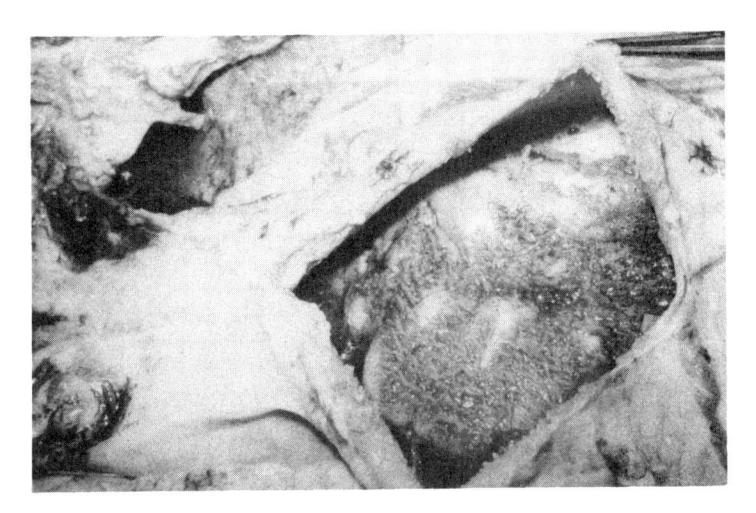

Figure 3.2

267. The diagnosis most likely is

    (A) miliary tuberculosis
    (B) candidemia
    (C) viral pericarditis
    (D) fibrinous pericarditis
    (E) mesothelioma

268. Treatment for this condition would be

    (A) pericardiocentesis
    (B) intracavitary steroid injection
    (C) pericardial window
    (D) pericardiectomy
    (E) amphotericin B

269. The congestive failure is due to

    (A) low output
    (B) high pulmonary vascular resistance
    (C) myocardiopathy
    (D) valvular stenosis
    (E) low filling pressure

ANSWERS AND TUTORIAL ON ITEMS 267-269

The answers are: **267-D; 268-D; 269-A**.

This patient has uremic fibrinous pericarditis. Because of the encasement of the pericardium, only a very low filling on venous return is possible and the patient experiences low output congestive failure. Treatment for this would not be instillation of anything into the pericardium, so much as relief of the "coeurasse" encasing the heart. The myocardium is adequate to function if it had a filling volume of blood it could eject, but fibrinous pericarditis is a restriction of the cardiac output based in this limitation on venous filling. Early in the disease, a pericardial "window" allows drainage of this uremic pericarditis; however, late in the development in which fibrinous pericarditis occurs and the pericardial sac stiffens to become an encasement, this restrictive pericarditis on the basis of its fibrinous nature is best treated by pericardiectomy.

ESRD → uremic fibrinous pericarditis
- very low filling on venous return
- low output CHF

Tx: pericardial window, pericardiectomy

Items 270-272

A 46 year-old man confined to his hospital bed after an orthopedic injury in an car accident develops deep venous thrombosis. He has one episode of pleuritic chest pain and hemoptysis and is anticoagulated, but 2 days later develops tachypnea and an X-ray is shown in **Figure 3.3**.

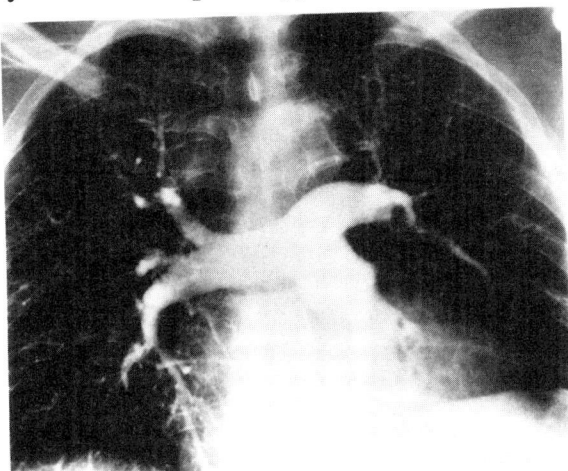

Figure 3.3

270. Indications for surgical intervention for thromboembolism include each of the following **EXCEPT**:

    (A) pulmonary angiographic evidence
    (B) patient having had 5,000 units heparin b.i.d.
    (C) recurrent pulmonary emboli
    (D) full therapeutic anticoagulation
    (E) contraindication to full heparinization (e.g., closed head injury)

271. In the X-ray seen, the patient has

    (A) main pulmonary arterial stenosis
    (B) left lung defect
    (C) right lung defect
    (D) saddle embolus
    (E) bilateral emboli

272. Treatment for this specific embolus might include

    (A) transvenous umbrella
    (B) caval clipping
    (C) coumadin
    (D) urokinase infusion
    (E) heparin anticoagulation

ANSWERS AND TUTORIAL ON ITEMS 270-272

The answers are: **270-B; 271-E; 272-D**.

This pulmonary angiogram demonstrates bilateral pulmonary emboli through the cut-offs seen on the pulmonary end-arteries. Surgical means of treatment of pulmonary emboli or interruption of the next embolus before it reaches the lungs are based on *angiographic* evidence of *recurrent* pulmonary emboli on full *therapeutic* anticoagulation or in the presence of *contraindications* thereto. This means that full therapeutic anticoagulation is a necessary antecedent, and not the "mini-dose" heparin that is not anticoagulating, but does have some protective benefit in reducing the incidence of deep venous thrombosis and pulmonary emboli.

Each of the treatments for pulmonary embolus that are recommended such as transvenous umbrella, caval clipping, coumadin or heparin relate to the *next* embolus. It is urokinase infusion that relates to the embolus already present in the lung to hasten its fibrinolysis. The only directed surgical attempt at treatment of the pulmonary embolus already sustained is the so-called Trendelenburg operation in which pulmonary arteriotomy is performed and the clot is "milked" back out of the lungs in which it is lodged. This is a very major operation requiring cardiopulmonary bypass and is rarely indicated, since patients who survive to the point of getting to the operating room for such an operation are likely going to survive with full systemic heparinization and thrombolytic therapy. The majority of the patients who suffer sudden lethal pulmonary embolus have it as a saddle embolus which gives rise to rapid right heart strain and fibrillation. Such patients would be unlikely to benefit from operation which could not be mobilized in time to be of benefit.

Items 273-275

A 51 year-old man had cough, weight loss and blood tinged sputum develop over 6 months and a chest X-ray is done. The results show a finding depicted in **Figure 3.4**.

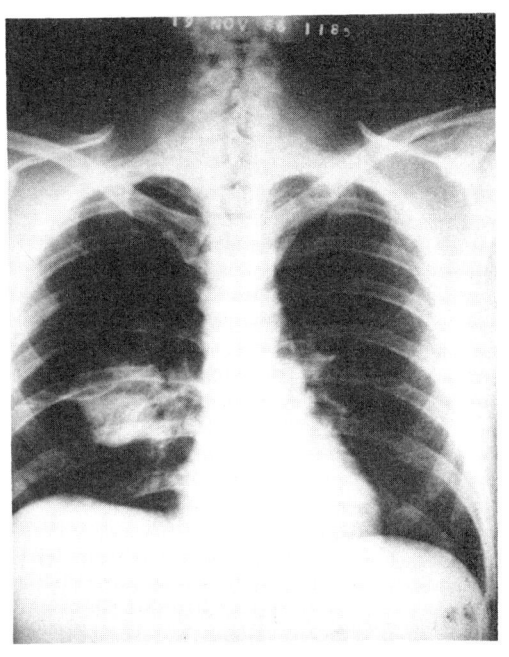

Figure 3.4

273. The next step in diagnosis is

    (A)   percutaneous aspiration cytology
    (B)   thoracentesis
    (C)   pulmonary function studies
    (D)   mediastinoscopy
    (E)   bronchoscopy

274. With the diagnosis of anaplastic carcinoma, the next step is

    (A)   pulmonary function tests
    (B)   thoracentesis
    (C)   mediastinoscopy
    (D)   thoracotomy
    (E)   chemotherapy

275. If the patient has reasonable pulmonary reserve, what determines resectability for this anaplastic carcinoma?

   (A)   cell type
   (B)   malignant pleural effusion
   (C)   positive mediastinoscopic nodes
   (D)   chest wall invasion
   (E)   positive cervical nodes

ANSWERS AND TUTORIAL ON ITEMS 273-275

The answers are: **273-E; 274-E; 275-A**.

This patient has anaplastic carcinoma of the right middle lobe. Although it presents as a coin lesion, it is usually widely disseminated and unlikely to be resectable. The nonresectability of this lesion even in a patient who is operable is based on its cell type rather than any specific contraindication, since this disease is better treated with chemotherapy than by futile extensive resection. The purpose of the bronchoscopy is to establish the diagnosis, and thereafter appropriate therapy can be planned and initiated.

Items 276-278

A coal miner had been PPD skin test positive and had an interval series of chest X-rays to check for evidence of black lung. On one such examination (**Figure 3.5A**), a finding was noted that progressed in 9 months (**Figure 3.5B**) and at one year (**Figure 3.5C** and **D**).

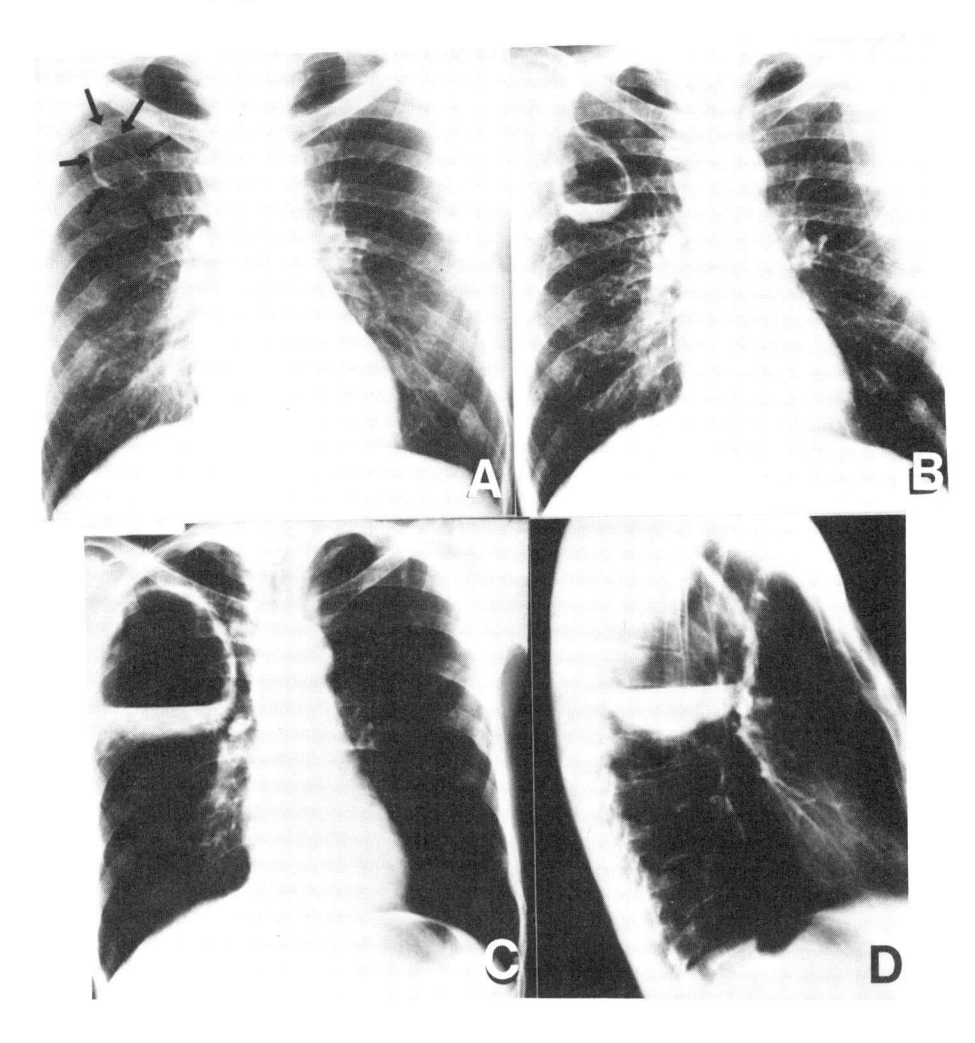

Figure 3.5

276. The next best treatment should be

    (A)   pneumonectomy
    (B)   bronchoscopy and brush biopsy
    (C)   postural drainage
    (D)   tube thoracostomy
    (E)   percutaneous aspiration

277. The likely reason for the significant change in this lesion is

   (A) resistant mycobacteria
   (B) malignancy
   (C) pyogenic abscess
   (D) fungal superinfection
   (E) bronchopleural fistula

278. Helpful pre-operative tests of operability would include

   (A) pulmonary function tests
   (B) arterial P_{CO_2}
   (C) thoracentesis
   (D) trans-tracheal aspiration
   (E) pulmonary CT

ANSWERS AND TUTORIAL ON ITEMS 276-278

The answers are: **276-B; 277-B; 278-A**.

This patient has progression of a cavitary lesion that probably began as tuberculosis. Because of the cavitation of this pulmonary abscess, and also because of the unknown nature of the lesion, bronchoscopy and brush biopsy would be recommended. The brush biopsy would give histologic evidence of the nature of the lesion as well as open up the abscess into the bronchi for the possibility of postural drainage and evacuation of the collection that is partially aerated suggesting communication with the bronchus. Although various superinfections and other problems may take place in such a lesion, the most significant one in this instance proven by the brush biopsy is a malignant degeneration.

Whether this patient can be operated on would be a determination assisted by the results of his pulmonary function tests. Abnormal arterial P_{CO_2} is a very late finding in a chronic pulmonary cripple, and the other tests listed relate largely to resectability of the tumor rather than operability of the patient.

Items 279-282

      (A)   Superficial thrombophlebitis
      (B)   Deep venous thrombosis
      (C)   Both
      (D)   Neither

279. pulmonary embolus

280. occult visceral malignancy

281. heparin therapy

282. early ambulation reduces likelihood

ANSWERS AND TUTORIAL ON ITEMS 279-282

The answers are: **279-B; 280-A; 281-C; 282-B**.

    The biggest threat from deep venous thrombosis is dislodging and embolizing the clot which may migrate to the lungs. This would be unlikely to occur with superficial thrombophlebitis, which is above the fascia through which perforating veins carry superficial venous return to the deep venous system or through the saphenous collecting system. Migratory superficial thrombophlebitis that is otherwise unexplained may be a harbinger of malignancy, particularly in neoplasms that are associated with a hypercoaguable state.

    Heparin therapy is useful in both. Low dose heparin is used for prevention and therapeutic anticoagulation levels for treatment, which do not so much dissolve the clots as prevent coagulation and any propagation as the thrombolytic system works on clot lysis. Early ambulation enlists the assistance of muscular contraction to minimize stasis, pumping blood up to the next higher venous valve enroute to the heart. The superficial venous system is external to the fascia enveloping the muscles, and would not experience compression from muscular exertion. Locally applied heat might increase blood flow through the superficial venous system, but muscular pumping would be on the opposite side of the fascial barrier, and if the perforating veins have competent valves, that pressure would not be translated to the superficial venous system.

Items 283-286

      (A) Open pneumothorax
      (B) Tension pneumothorax
      (C) Both
      (D) Neither

283. interferes with airflow in opposite lung

284. survivable in absence of emergency treatment

285. impairs cardiac output

286. dyspnea

ANSWERS AND TUTORIAL ON ITEMS 283-286

The answers are: **283-B; 284-A; 285-B; 286-C**.

Open pneumothorax interferes with airflow in the lung on the affected side due to the portion of lung that has collapsed, but does not appreciably interfere with ventilation of the opposite side. Because of the shift in the mediastinum from the air trapped in the pleural space under tension, tension pneumothorax compromises the ventilatory function of the opposite lung as well. This pressure of accumulated intrathoracic air also interferes with venous return, and impairs cardiac output, an effect only minimally possible with open pneumothorax which should have no additional effect beyond the loss of negative intrathoracic pressure that may help in venous return in the closed chest.

Dyspnea is a feature of both conditions, with the sucking sound of an open pneumothorax creating high anxiety in the patient so afflicted. However, since tension pneumothorax is not survivable without emergency treatment and open pneumothorax is, an emergency method of management would be to convert the tension pneumothorax into an open one, and that is the definitive medical treatment as well when that open pneumothorax is controlled by tube thoracostomy to a water seal.

Items 287-290

        (A)   Lobectomy
        (B)   Pneumonectomy
        (C)   Both
        (D)   Neither

287. occasionally used in tuberculosis treatment

288. operable patient can climb only two flights pre-operatively

289. required for stage IV lung carcinoma

290. chest tube not necessary

ANSWERS AND TUTORIAL ON ITEMS 287-290

The answers are: **287-A; 288-A; 289-D; 290-B**.

    Pulmonary resection is an operation based on recommendations of resectability and operability with a view to improved postoperative function. The rule of thumb has been that a patient who can walk one flight of stairs without stopping can undergo thoracotomy, two flights of stairs lobectomy, and three flights of stairs pneumonectomy. This simple rule of thumb is as close an approximation to quick and inexpensive pulmonary function testing as can be obtained in practical circumstances. So, a patient who cannot climb (based on pulmonary insufficiency) a third flight of stairs is inoperable if the lesion requires pneumonectomy for resection. A tumor, therefore, resectable by pneumonectomy in this inoperable patient would mean that such an operation should not be undertaken, since the patient would be a pulmonary cripple who could not survive without ventilator therapy even if that brief survival were tumor free. Neither lobectomy nor pneumonectomy would be adequate resection for stage IV lung cancer, and would not be recommended, let alone required.

    Lobectomy is occasionally used for the cavitary destruction of a lobe which has not collapsed with the encouragement of endoscopic drainage. Tuberculosis, it is granted, is not an anatomically confined disease but may be spread more widely through the lungs, bilaterally at that. But the surgical treatment is not that of tuberculosis but of a complication of tuberculosis, since it is presumed that the tuberculosis is treated with chemotherapy and the architectural unresolved problem in the lobe may be resected. Because tuberculosis is a pneumonia, it usually leaves some degree of impairment in pulmonary function in the scarred healing process. It is unlikely, therefore, that pneumonectomy would be a treatment for a complication of tuberculosis, since the opposite lung that would have to support the patient would have some degree of disease if the tuberculous complication that is present in one side of the chest is so extensive as to require total pneumonectomy.

When total pneumonectomy is performed, a chest tube is not required, whereas it is for lobectomy, in which evacuation of the pleural air is performed in order to allow expansion of the lung that remains to fill the pleural space. Since there is no lung remaining after total pneumonectomy, fibrothorax is anticipated, and the fluid and air in the pleural space left at the time of closure are not evacuated.

Items 291-294

(A) Coarctation of aorta
(B) Aneurysm of abdominal aorta
(C) Both
(D) Neither

291. congenital

292. acute dissection

293. antihypertensive therapy

294. cardiopulmonary bypass

ANSWERS AND TUTORIAL ON ITEMS 291-294

The answers are: **291-A; 292-B; 293-C; 294-D**.

Coarctation is a constriction of the aorta and is congenital; aneurysm is a dilatation of the aorta and is usually acquired. Both are associated with hypertension, the former because coarctation is a cause of hypertension. The latter often has hypertension associated with it, and antihypertensive therapy is often used in management of aneurysm, particularly in conservative follow-up of those aneurysms that have not reached size thought to be a threat for dissection. When expansion or dissection occurs, antihypertensive treatment can be employed as an emergency, lowering the pressure head on the dissecting aorta which might recanalize into a "double barrel", and if there is no compromise to visceral organ function (particularly the kidneys or gut) elective aneurysm resection can be carried out rather than an emergency operation for the dissection. Cardiopulmonary bypass would be needed for neither instance of operation on the abdominal aorta. Thoracic arch aneurysm resection has a different clinical disease pattern, and it may be repaired, frequently employing cardiopulmonary bypass for repair of aortic arch aneurysm.

Items 295-298

(A) Tension pneumothorax
(B) Pericardial tamponade
(C) Both
(D) Neither

295. interferes with venous return to the heart

296. jugular venous distension

297. survival likely if untreated

298. needle aspiration both diagnostic and therapeutic

ANSWERS AND TUTORIAL ON ITEMS 295-298

The answers are: **295-C; 296-C; 297-D; 298-C**.

Tension pneumothorax and pericardial tamponade are both collections of fluid under pressure that interfere with a normal fluid flow in and out of thoracic cavities. In the case of tension pneumothorax, the fluid trapped under pressure is air and the principle disturbance is to the flow of air in and out of not only the affected lung, but also the opposite side. In the case of pericardial tamponade, the fluid trapped outside the circulation is blood and it is in the pericardium rather than the air in the pleura, with an interference in venous return that compromises cardiac output.

However, both "tensions" also interfere with blood flow, impeding venous return to the heart by abolishing the changes in intrathoracic pressure that is negative on the inspiratory cycle of normal respiration. Therefore, jugular venous distension occurs in both and cardiac output impairment occurs with both. Needle aspiration of the pleura and the pericardium is both diagnostic and therapeutic in each. It is also necessary, since survival in each circumstance is very unlikely if untreated, and each is an emergency that should be managed immediately once recognized.

Items 299-303

(A) Chronic bronchitis
(B) Emphysema
(C) Asthma
(D) Tuberculosis
(E) Pneumoconiosis
(F) Cystic fibrosis

299. Treatment with epinephrine.

300. Most common cause of fixed "barrel chest".

301. Pneumothorax once was used for treatment.

302. Silo fillers may experience one type of this condition.

303. Decreased reproductive potential.

ANSWERS AND TUTORIAL ON ITEMS 299-303

The answers are: **299-C; 300-B; 301-D; 302-E; 303-F**.

Of the chronic lung diseases listed, asthma is primarily of the bronchoconstrictive variety and treatment with epinephrine infusion is appropriate for asthma and not for the other conditions. Hyperinflation and difficulty with incomplete exhalation is characteristic of emphysema, and over time, the hyperinflated chest expansion becomes fixed in the "barrel chest" deformity. Of the inflammatory lung diseases that leads to fibrosis, one is a peculiar occupational hazard related to inhalation of oxides of nitrogen in the process of silage decomposition. Inhalation of these oxides can result in acid injury to the lungs, and this silo fillers' disease is one form of pneumoconiosis.

Pneumothorax, not as complication, but as treatment, was employed at one time for tuberculosis. This took the form of phrenic nerve crush, or stuffing the chest with masses that could deflate the lung such as ping-pong balls; eventually this pneumothorax has given way to thoracoplasty in which the lung is not collapsed within the chest as much as the chest is brought down to the lung. These forms of late-stage tuberculosis treatment, fortunately, are now rare with better antimicrobial chemotherapy, but with the emerging resistance in high risk patient groups, it may be too early to describe these forms of therapy as obsolete.

Cystic fibrosis is described also by another name mucoviscidosis. Not only is this a disease of pulmonary secretory epithelium, but it also effects secretory epithelium everywhere giving rise to problems in the gut, pancreas, and in germ cell production as well. Reproductive potential is impaired in this epithelial defect.

Items 304-308

(A) Mitral stenosis
(B) Mitral insufficiency
(C) Aortic stenosis
(D) Coronary insufficiency

304. Most common chronic cardiac consequence of rheumatic fever.

305. Source of migratory pulmonary abscesses in addicts.

306. (Stokes-Adams) syncopal attacks.

307. Characteristic jugular venous pulsation.

308. Lowering diastolic blood pressure may result in symptoms.

ANSWERS AND TUTORIAL ON ITEMS 304-308

The answers are: **304-A; 305-A; 306-C; 307-B; 308-D.**

Mitral stenosis is a common cardiac consequence of rheumatic fever, and with the decrease in rheumatic fever (presumably because of the reduction in streptococcal valvular disease from the ubiquitous administration of penicillin in childhood) rheumatic mitral stenosis has been decreasing in the United States. If acute valvulitis occurs as may be the case with illicit drug and excipient debris injected into the venous circulation, right heart vegetations can give rise to migratory pulmonary abscesses, which is radiographic evidence of IV drug abuse. Insufficiency of the mitral valve would give venous regurgitation, being evident on clinical exam in jugular venous pulses.

At the level of the aortic valve, stenosis may give rise to transient attacks of ischemia in the carotid circulation, and these acute ischemic episodes give syncopal or Stokes-Adams attacks. This is a very dangerous threat to neurologic function. The aorta has as its first branches from the sinuses beyond the aortic valve the coronary artery ostia. The coronaries are perfused with diastolic blood pressure, since the maximum blood flow occurs when the aortic valve is closed and the coronary ostia are open to perfusion at maximum flows. Therefore, lowering the diastolic blood pressure may result in symptomatic coronary insufficiency.

Items 309-313

(A) Radiolabeled ^{131}I fibrinogen
(B) Venogram
(C) Plethysmography
(D) Doppler flow scan
(E) Pulmonary arteriogram

309. The definitive accurate test of deep venous thrombosis.

310. Required before surgical treatment of thromboembolism is considered.

311. Can localize future blood clot but not those that have already been formed.

312. A noninvasive test that does not require complete obstruction for detection of clot.

313. The test with the highest risk of communicable disease transmission.

ANSWERS AND TUTORIAL ON ITEMS 309-313

The answers are: **309-B; 310-E; 311-A; 312-A; 313-A.**

The "gold standard" of deep venous thrombosis diagnosis is venography. However, it is invasive to the degree that it causes some degree of venous inflammation that may even lead to deep venous thrombosis if none were present before the test. Therefore, alternatives to this best study are sought, and several noninvasive methods are proposed. Fibrinogen that is radiolabeled can determine clot formation without complete obstruction. However, it only localizes blood clot prospectively and does not identify that which has already been formed. It also has a disadvantage in that it is the test of those listed with the highest risk of transmission of communicable disease, since it is a plasma-derived product.

Before surgical treatment of thromboembolism is considered, pulmonary angiographic evidence of recurrent pulmonary embolism on adequate anticoagulation therapy or with major contraindications thereto must be confirmed. Medical treatment of thromboembolism does not have these requirements, and it is the primary therapy of thromboembolism, not limited to recurrent disease that is not only present in the deep veins of the lower extremities but has also migrated by angiographic proof to the lungs.

Items 314-318

    (A)   Low dose heparin
    (B)   High dose heparin anticoagulation
    (C)   Caval filtration umbrella
    (D)   Operative caval clip application
    (E)   Ligation inferior vena cava
    (F)   Ligation left ovarian vein
    (G)   Venous thrombectomy
    (H)   Pulmonary embolectomy (Trendelenburg procedure)

314. A widely applicable method of thromboembolism prevention.

315. An operation for risk reduction that has no application outside the iliac area.

316. A percutaneous means of preventing the next thromboembolism.

317. Adequate therapy for most patients with deep venous thrombosis.

318. A last salvage procedure after recurrent pulmonary embolism in patients who have been on full anticoagulation.

ANSWERS AND TUTORIAL ON ITEMS 314-318

The answers are: **314-A; 315-G; 316-C; 317-B; 318-H**.

Low dose heparin (5000 Units subcutaneously q 12 hours) is widely applicable, since it can be employed in patients who are unable to ambulate or cooperate in the other measures of thromboembolism prevention. It does not require monitoring, since this dose of heparin therapy is not anticoagulating. Venous thrombectomy should in theory be appropriate as a procedure to reduce thromboembolism risk by removing the thrombus. However, it has no role in any area outside the iliac veins where it is quite limited in application as well. The better means of removing thrombus would be by thrombolytic process, and that occurs without invasion of the vein and the potential for suture line or other endothelial interruption and new clot formation on the nidus of local inflammation.

Most surgical therapy of thromboembolism is directed at the prevention of the next thromboemboli migrating to the lung, and intercepting them in the cava. A percutaneous method of accomplishing this is by the introduction of caval filters (Mobin-Uddin, Greenfield). This same means is applied, frequently as accessory to operation in which the caval area is already exposed, through application of a clip or other compartmentalization procedure. Most patients who have deep venous thrombosis are adequately treated by full anticoagulation high dose heparin therapy. This allows the natural process of clot lysis to occur while preventing the formation of new thrombus.

The final salvage procedure in some patients might be those who have suffered recurrent pulmonary embolism that has used up the last of their marginal reserves and put them into acute right heart failure despite full anticoagulation therapy. This is the Trendelenburg procedure which requires full cardiopulmonary bypass in its performance and is a very major undertaking with very low probability of survival in most patients who would be most in need of it.

Items 319-328

319. Which of the following suggests unresectability of a left upper lobe lung cancer?

    (A) hemoptysis
    (B) pneumonia
    (C) malignant pleural effusion
    (D) a cough specimen with positive sputum cytology
    (E) clubbing and blueness of fingers

320. Management of pulmonary complications of tuberculosis refractory to antibiotic management include each of the following **EXCEPT**:

    (A) decortication
    (B) chest wall reconstruction
    (C) hyperbaric oxygen therapy
    (D) bronchoscopic brush biopsy and lavage
    (E) lobectomy

321. Which of the following associated conditions indicates dissemination of small cell carcinoma of the lung?

    (A) Cushing's syndrome
    (B) myasthenic (Eaton-Lambert) syndrome
    (C) superior sulcus syndrome
    (D) hypertrophic pulmonary osteoarthropathy
    (E) polycythemia

322. Which of the following is **LEAST** likely as a diagnosis when a left upper lobe "coin lesion" is discovered on the chest X-ray screening of an asymptomatic 40 year-old white male?

    (A) sarcoidosis
    (B) hamartoma
    (C) adenocarcinoma
    (D) squamous cell carcinoma
    (E) tuberculosis

323. *Pneumocystis carinii* pneumonia

    (A) occurs only in patients who are HIV-positive
    (B) begins as a perihilar infiltrate pattern on chest X-ray
    (C) responds to erythromycin
    (D) usually presents as a productive cough
    (E) only rarely causes severe hypoxia

324. A 54 year-old man with a "barreled chest" undergoes mediastinoscopy for staging of lung cancer identified by a positive sputum cytology. Hilar lymph node biopsy has shown frozen section histology negative for tumor. Three hours following mediastinoscopy the patient is in dyspneic crisis with a cyanotic dusky complexion and fearful expression with neck veins distended. You should immediately

    (A) order chest X-ray
    (B) insert large bore needle in both sides of the chest
    (C) ventilate with ambulatory manual breathing unit (AMBU) bag
    (D) place a bag over patient's nose and mouth for rebreathing
    (E) perform tracheotomy

325. Cyanosis is a prominent clinical feature of each of the following conditions **EXCEPT**:

    (A) *cor pulmonale*
    (B) tetralogy of Fallot
    (C) aortic stenosis
    (D) pulmonary atresia
    (E) tricuspid stenosis

326. Pulmonary artery banding in children is indicated in which of the following conditions?

    (A) large ventricular septal defect
    (B) coarctation of the aorta
    (C) "pink" tetralogy of Fallot
    (D) distal pulmonary atresia
    (E) aortic stenosis

327. The most frequently performed procedure for coronary insufficiency currently is

    (A) internal mammary artery bypass
    (B) coronary endarterectomy
    (C) coronary thrombectomy
    (D) aortocoronary bypass graft
    (E) percutaneous coronary angioplasty

328. Satisfactory methods of treating mitral valve disease include each of the following **EXCEPT**:

    (A) mitral commissurotomy (Harken)
    (B) xenograft valve prosthesis (Carpentier-Edwards)
    (C) tilting disk mitral valve prosthesis (Bjork-Shiley)
    (D) ball valve prosthesis (Starr-Edwards)
    (E) aortic homograft prosthesis

ANSWERS AND TUTORIALS ON ITEMS 319-328

The answers are: **319-C; 320-C; 321-C; 322-A; 323-B; 324-B; 325-C; 326-A; 327-D; 328-C**.

319. Pneumonia, hemoptysis and clubbing are all signs that may be related to benign pulmonary disease as well as resectable malignancy, and positive sputum cytology on cough specimen does not rule out resection for cure since it is presumed to originate from the cancer already identified in the left upper lobe. If the cytology were from a catheter transbronchial aspirant from the right lung, it would suggest bilateral disease making this patient with clubbing and pneumonia inoperable as well as suggesting a tumor that is nonresectable. The single contraindication to operation planned for resection for cure is the positive finding of a malignant pleural effusion, since this indicates that the cancer has spread beyond the confines of the lobe and would not be cured even by left pneumonectomy.

320. Tuberculosis can result in local destruction of affected lung with cavitation. If this cavitary destruction is large, if it is multiple in one lobe, and if it is not successfully drained intrabronchially through the assistance of bronchoscopic brush biopsy to enter the cavity and lavage, lobectomy may be advised. A thickened pleura is likely, particularly if a secondary bacterial infection and empyema result which may require thorough drainage of the pleural space and decortication of the encased lung in order to allow expansion. If that expansion is not possible with the lung coming up to the chest wall, the chest wall is actually collapsed down onto the lung, in a type of chest wall reconstruction called thoracoplasty. Each of these surgical methods has been used with success with management of complications of tuberculosis. Hyperbaric oxygen therapy is not successful in managing these complications.

321. Small cell carcinoma of the lung is associated with several paraneoplastic syndromes. Myasthenia symptoms, like those of myasthenia gravis, are described in the Eaton-Lambert syndrome. ACTH-like endocrine responses can be seen with a Cushinoid appearance. Both polycythemia and an unusual form of osteoarthropathy involving sub-periosteal growth suggests messengers with erythropoietin-like or growth hormone-like activity. Each of these are secondary to physiologic responses, and polycythemia may be a response to chronic desaturation even without the presence of an excess peptide mediator postulated. However, superior sulcus syndrome is a phenomenon of malignant obstruction to the innominate venous return and superior sympathetic chain, and indicates metastatic disease outside the confines of the lung.

322. Sarcoidosis is found in younger age groups predominately, and as a rule it does not present as a solitary "coin lesion". It is also higher in incidence in African-American than in Caucasian patients. Adenocarcinoma may present in this fashion in the lung, and is probably more likely to represent metastatic disease than primary pulmonary adenocarcinoma. The fortunate but rare benign tumor known as hamartoma presents as a "coin lesion", but unfortunately the more common "coin lesion" encountered radiographically, even on screening asymptomatic patients, is squamous cell carcinoma. Tuberculosis may present as a solitary lesion, before cavitation in the later stages when communication with the bronchus occurs in later stages of caseation. These lesions are all primary pulmonary lesions and sarcoidosis is more likely to be perihilar in position and involving mediastinal lymphatic structures as a rule.

323. One of the earliest presentations for *Pneumocystis* is a nonproductive cough. Because of the interstitial location of the protozoa, sputum production is remarkably absent. In such patients rapid and severe hypoxia and desaturation occur early; and, as the major morbid feature, out of proportion to clinical findings on auscultation. Chest X-ray early in such patients shows perihilar infiltrate in a "butterfly" pattern, progressive to later consolidation. The protozoan does not respond to erythromycin antibiotic as *Mycoplasma* or *Legionella* often do. *Pneumocystis* occurs in patients who have been immunocompromised. This includes, but is not limited to, patients infected with HIV . Earlier cases of *Pneumocystis* showed a predominance among premature malnourished infants, lymphoma patients under chemotherapy, or patients immunosuppressed for transplantation.

324. Mediastinoscopy is a valuable staging procedure for identifying potential spread from lung cancer. In a patient with chronic disease, the mediastinum may be displaced by intrapleural expansion. Both mediastinoscopy and node biopsy may result in entry into the pleura that can be unrecognized at the time of the procedure, and the ventilation of the patient during the operation can result in a ruptured emphysematous bleb. The patient's clinical condition is nearly instantly recognizable as tension pneumothorax. There is no time for chest X-ray, and especially not if the patient is sent away to a radiography suite for it, out of an environment of higher nursing intensity. The symptoms are not suggestive of upper airway obstruction, and if hematoma or other compression were obstructing the lower trachea or bronchi, tracheotomy would be above this obstruction and would serve no purpose in relief of it. AMBU bag ventilation is contraindicated, since this would serve to further insufflate air under tension higher than that which a patient is already experiencing from the intrapleural air accumulation through the ventilatory effort. Clinical exam which would consist of listening to each side of the chest might suggest which side to begin, but thoracostomy is urgently indicated. One of the safest and quickest ways to carry this out is with a large bore needle on a 50 ml syringe. Inserting this in the pleural space of each side of the chest, the side most suspicious by clinical examination first, causes the plunger to jump from the barrel of the syringe on the side with tension pneumothorax, simultaneously diagnosing and relieving the patient's inhalatory emergency until longer term management can proceed through placement of tube thoracostomy.

325. Malformation of the tricuspid valve (Ebstein's deformity) causes reduction in right ventricular output, and, hence, cyanosis. The same is true for reduction in pulmonary flow in the shunting seen in the tetralogy of Fallot and pulmonary atresia. An increase in pulmonary vascular resistance as in *cor pulmonale* also constitutes a pulmonary arterial flow restriction, and each of these reductions in pulmonary arterial blood flow is associated with cyanosis. Aortic stenosis, however, should not affect hemodynamics or oxygen saturation in the right circulation, but is a problem in the perfusion of blood from the left side of the heart that has already been oxygenated, so cyanosis is absent.

326. High volume left to right shunt can give refractory congestive failure in patients too ill or too small to undergo total surgical correction. Temporary palliation may be achieved by diminishing pulmonary artery pressure through a constriction of the pulmonary trunk. This would hardly be necessary in a patient who already had an atretic segment of pulmonary artery. The patient with pink tetralogy is manifesting compensation whereby congestive failure is not prominent from left to right shunt. In the classic operation for cyanotic tetralogy, pulmonary blood flow and pressure was actually increased to early systolic systemic levels by creating a fistula through the subclavian artery diversion (Blalock-Taussig) or aortopulmonary window anastomosis (Waterston). This is the reverse of the pressure dynamics attempted with a pulmonary banding procedure.

Both coarctation of the aorta and valve stenosis are, in effect, "banding" of the left ventricular outflow, causing some degree of left heart strain, and pulmonary banding would not address any therapeutic purpose in lowering a normal pulmonary arterial pressure besides creating additional right ventricular strain. Only the patient with significant congestive failure from refractory pulmonary hypertension that cannot undergo total anatomic correction should undergo this palliative procedure, and with improvements in both medical management of pulmonary hypertension and earlier definitive repair, the palliative pulmonary banding procedure is becoming much less commonly indicated.

327. Thrombectomy for coronary artery thrombosis is as temporary as coronary endarterectomy, both of which do not improve blood flow long-term and, hence, myocardial performance. The Vineberg internal mammary artery bypass was useful when originally proposed and remains so for selected indications, but the majority of patients today undergo bypass grafting from aorta to coronary arteries through reversed saphenous veins or some other conduit than the internal mammary artery. Percutaneous transcatheter coronary angioplasty might be applicable to patients with isolated lesions, but most coronary atherosclerosis is generalized with not just a single focal significant stenotic lesion, so even patients with coronary angioplasty procedure are standby candidates for coronary artery bypass graft from aorta, which is the most frequently performed operation.

328. The repair of a stenotic valve in the mitral position can take the form of mitral commissurotomy to increase mobility of fused or stenotic mitral valve leaflets, although restenosis may be a long-term result. There is a dynamic tension between long-term recurrence of problems and low maintenance in adjunctive medication requirement with anticoagulation required for some prosthetic materials. Natural tissue seems to require less vigilance with respect to thrombotic problems which occur with less frequency with tissue, whether of xenograft or homograft origin, than with prosthetic synthetic materials. The ball valve design has been satisfactory if maintained with adequate anticoagulation, but the tilting disk has had an unacceptably high rate of dislocation, leading to embolization and sudden valvular insufficiency. For that reason, not only are those patients who require valve replacement not currently getting the option of tilting disk prosthesis, but there is a long-term recommendation for replacement of those already in place with a very low threshold for re-operation at the earliest sign of any symptoms.

CHAPTER IV
EMERGENCY AND TRAUMA SURGERY

Items 329-331

An apartment burglar is shot by police in an exchange of gunfire, and the left upper quadrant injury is explored revealing a wound in the left lateral lobe of the liver (**Figure 4.1**).

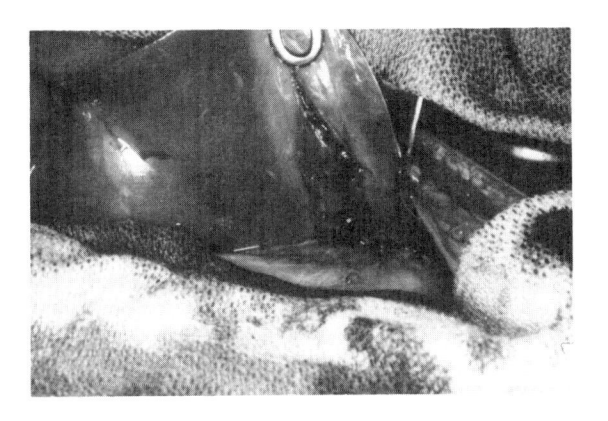

Figure 4.1

329. Treatment should be by

  (A) observing it
  (B) draining it
  (C) suturing it
  (D) resecting it
  (E) packing it

330. The clinically significant later component of this injury might likely be

  (A) loss of functioning liver
  (B) infection
  (C) leakage of bile
  (D) portal vein thrombosis
  (E) hemobilia

331. If he has no evident sequelae at 4 weeks he requires

 (A) follow-up arteriography
 (B) follow-up liver scan
 (C) CT
 (D) ultrasound
 (E) no specific follow-up

ANSWERS AND TUTORIAL ON ITEMS 329-331

The answers are: **329-D; 330-E; 331-E**.

The significant component of this penetrating injury is the perforation of the gut that lies behind the liver, in this case a through and through perforation of the stomach. This left lateral liver lobe injury may cause some peritoneal signs, but a more substantial component of liver is lost by a partial resection of this lobe. In suturing this lesion, as much liver would be defunctionalized and left *in situ* as would be removed in a relatively simple operation in removing this segment of the left lateral lobe. The significant component of that injury, therefore, is not so much the loss of liver or the risk of leakage or infection as the accumulation of any intrahepatic hematoma from some concomitant blunt injury from the deceleration of the missile. This intrahepatic liver hematoma can burst into the biliary tree and give the postoperative sequel of hemobilia. For that reason, the liver is searched for evidence of any blunt injury and hematoma following this penetrating wound. Follow-up of such patients is generally limited by the tolerance the patient has for making repeated medical visits, and often the patient is unavailable for follow-up by the same team of physicians if he is incarcerated in an institution. However, it is unlikely that he would require any specific follow-up if he were asymptomatic at 4 weeks following exploration.

Items 332-334

A burglary suspect was surprised by police upon exiting from a locked building, setting off an alarm. When he pulled out a weapon, he was shot in the abdomen at a range of 20 feet. The ileum is shown in **Figure 4.2** at laparotomy.

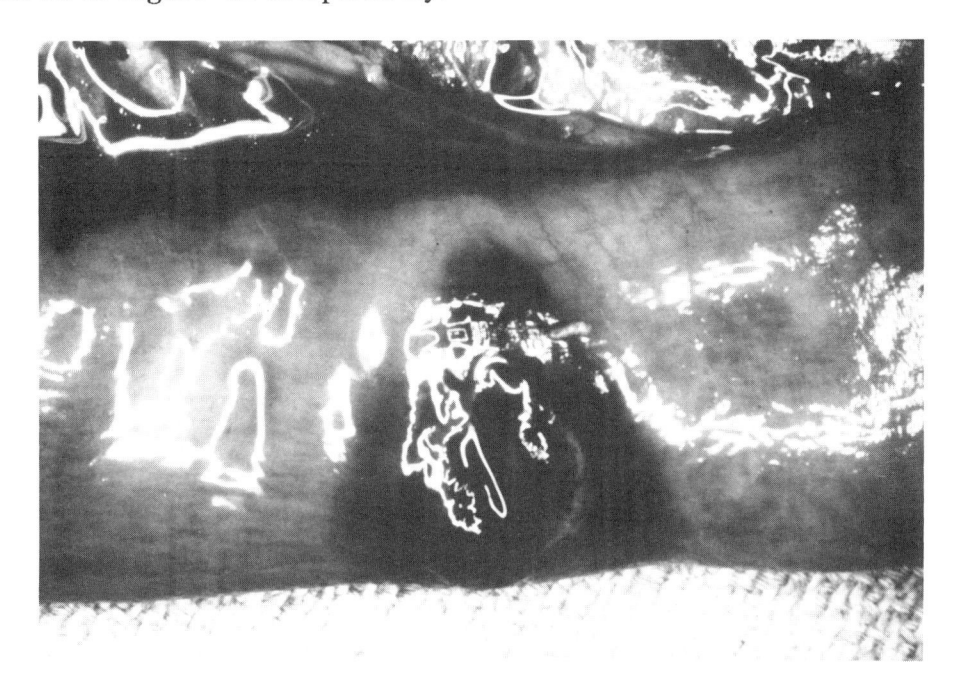

Figure 4.2

332. The weapon that caused this gunshot injury was

    (A)   low velocity handgun bullet
    (B)   high velocity handgun bullet
    (C)   shotgun
    (D)   high powered rifle
    (E)   hollow point bullet

333. The injury sustained can be described as

    (A)   blunt only
    (B)   penetrating only
    (C)   blunt and penetrating
    (D)   septic
    (E)   non-contaminated

334. Treatment should be by

   (A) simple closure of the hole
   (B) resection of the bowel segment
   (C) ileostomy
   (D) debridement and drainage
   (E) ileocolostomy

ANSWERS AND TUTORIAL ON ITEMS 332-334

The answers are: **332-A; 333-C; 334-B**.

This patient is injured by a police round. The objective of the handguns that police are issued is to instantly immobilize a personal threat to their own safety, and this is accomplished with a handgun with such power to immobilize the assailant, but not to assassinate him at some long range while he attempts to make an escape. This .38 calibre gunshot wound is found to have penetrated the abdomen and also to have perforated the bowel. But as can be clearly seen around the penetrating injury there is a rim of devitalized tissue, which had suffered from the shock of the passing missile. Its elastic limit has been exceeded and this area of the wound channel has been devitalized. This penetrating injury, therefore, had a blunt component, and other viscera not in the direct missile track (e.g., the spleen, nearby arteries that may have had intimal flaps raised in their disruption and other evidence of blunt and penetrating injury) must be examined for evidence of disruption. In the instance of this injury site, if a higher velocity weapon had been used, one might consider checking the chest viscera for blunt injury from the translation of higher velocity wound channels in the abdomen. The important feature here is to recognize that a penetrating injury of the viscera in the wound track may constitute a blunt injury to tissues outside the channel. For that reason, simple closure of perforation is inappropriate as treatment of what is obviously a penetrating wound without a recognition of the blunt component. The devitalized area of bowel around the perforation would have to be excised, and the probable method for doing so would be simple resection of this bowel segment.

Items 335-337

A 40 year-old worker for the gas company was investigating a complaint of a gas leak when an electrical short in a high voltage circuit nearby caused a spark ignition and explosion in the confined space where he was working. You see him in the ER on admission (**Figure 4.3**).

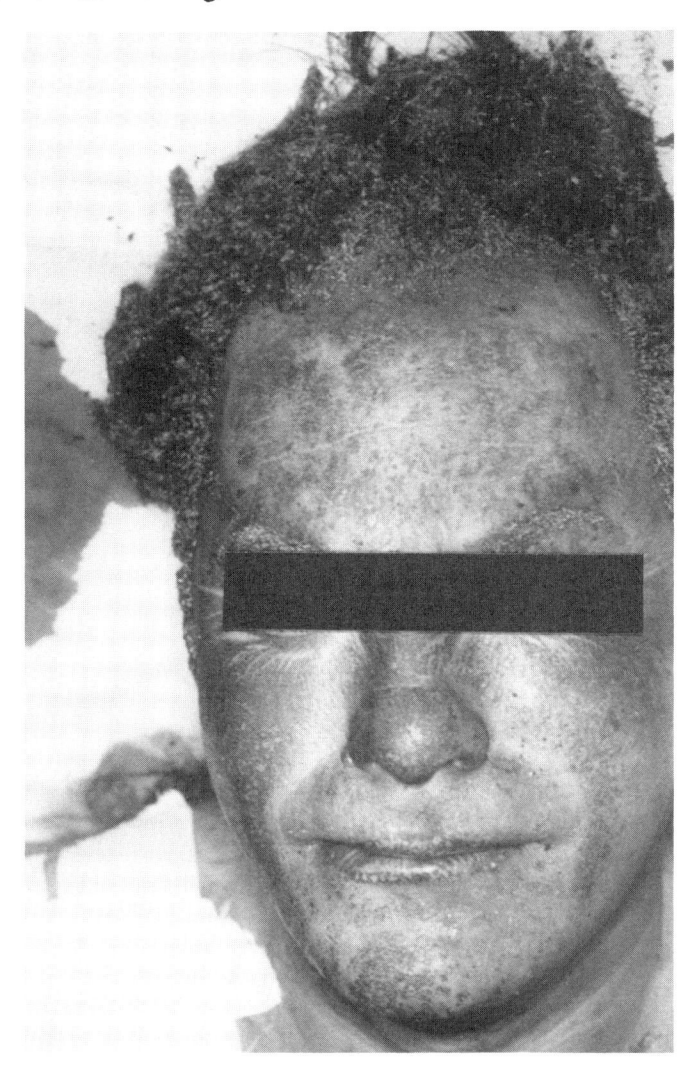

Figure 4.3

335. The chief concern at this point would be

    (A)   cosmetic result
    (B)   donor sites for grafting
    (C)   antibiotics for sepsis
    (D)   inhalation burn
    (E)   tetanus prophylaxis

336. The extent of the burn that is visible is probably

   (A)   9%
   (B)   18%
   (C)   1%
   (D)   36%
   (E)   54%

337. The depth and thickness of the burn visible is probably

   (A)   50% full thickness 50% partial thickness
   (B)   75% full thickness 25% partial thickness
   (C)   100% partial thickness
   (D)   100% full thickness
   (E)   it cannot be determined at this time

ANSWERS AND TUTORIAL ON ITEMS 335-337

The answers are: **335-D; 336-A; 337-E**.

This patient has suffered an explosion with a flash burn visible on the head. The frontal exposure that is seen here gives a 9% estimate as to the surface that is burned by the "rule of nines". However, the skin burn is indeterminate as far as the depth of the burn injury at this time, and the chief concern is not the skin burn or its subsequent cosmetic result or varying techniques of its management. The life-threatening injury in a flash burn with explosion is inhalation burn. The hot gases that resulted from the explosion would have been inhaled in the confined space. As a consequence, inhalation burn would be the single most urgent priority in this patient's management.

Items 338-340

A woman working in a laundry has her hand caught in a mangle. At the time of the emergency room visit (**Figure 4.4A**) the injury is depicted, and is seen again at two weeks (**Figure 4.4B**) when she returns for follow-up treatment.

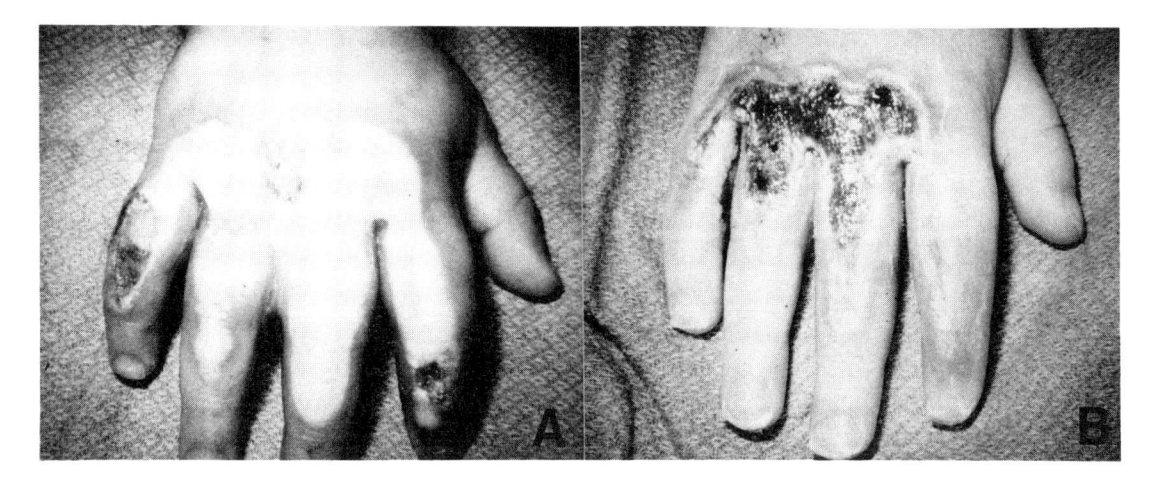

Figure 4.4

338. The first concern in the initial presentation would be

    (A) tetanus prophylaxis status
    (B) antibiotics for sepsis
    (C) evaluation of crush component of injury
    (D) immediate debridement of dead tissue
    (E) resurfacing with skin graft

339. As evident at 2 weeks, the proportion of the burn at original presentation was

    (A) 50% full thickness 50% partial thickness
    (B) 100% full thickness
    (C) 100% partial thickness
    (D) indeterminate even at 2 weeks
    (E) 90% full thickness 10% partial thickness

340. The most important endpoint in management of this injury will be

    (A) color match of graft with surrounding skin
    (B) coverage of extensor tendons
    (C) healed alignment of fractures
    (D) functional capability of the hand
    (E) minimized cosmetic soft tissue scarring

ANSWERS AND TUTORIAL ON ITEMS 338-340

The answers are: **338-C; 339-A; 340-D**.

This patient had the unfortunate combination of both thermal burn and mechanical injury to the hand, and injury in both bone and soft tissue components. On the initial evaluation, the burn injury is rather immediately apparent, although its extent in terms of depth is "declared" over time in observation. What is not immediately apparent but must be checked for at the time of presentation is the extent of the crush component of the injury. For that reason, X-ray of the hand should be obtained as well as a check on neurovascular components of each finger.

Over time, it is apparent that half of the burn wound was full thickness and half partial thickness, since the wound has shrunken about 50% of its original magnitude, which has happened faster than contraction could have taken place if the whole burn was originally full thickness tissue destruction of the skin of this hand.

The most important long-term objective in the management of hand injury generally is the functional capability of the hand. Whatever the hand looks like, so long as it functions well with limited disability, sacrifices in form and appearance would be made to maximize function. No cosmetically motivated treatment is acceptable that gives good appearance at a sacrifice of function in hand injury.

Items 341-343

A 35 year-old woman is involved as right front seat passenger in a head-on automobile collision. In the emergency room, she has a tender abdomen and has the appearance shown in **Figure 4.5**.

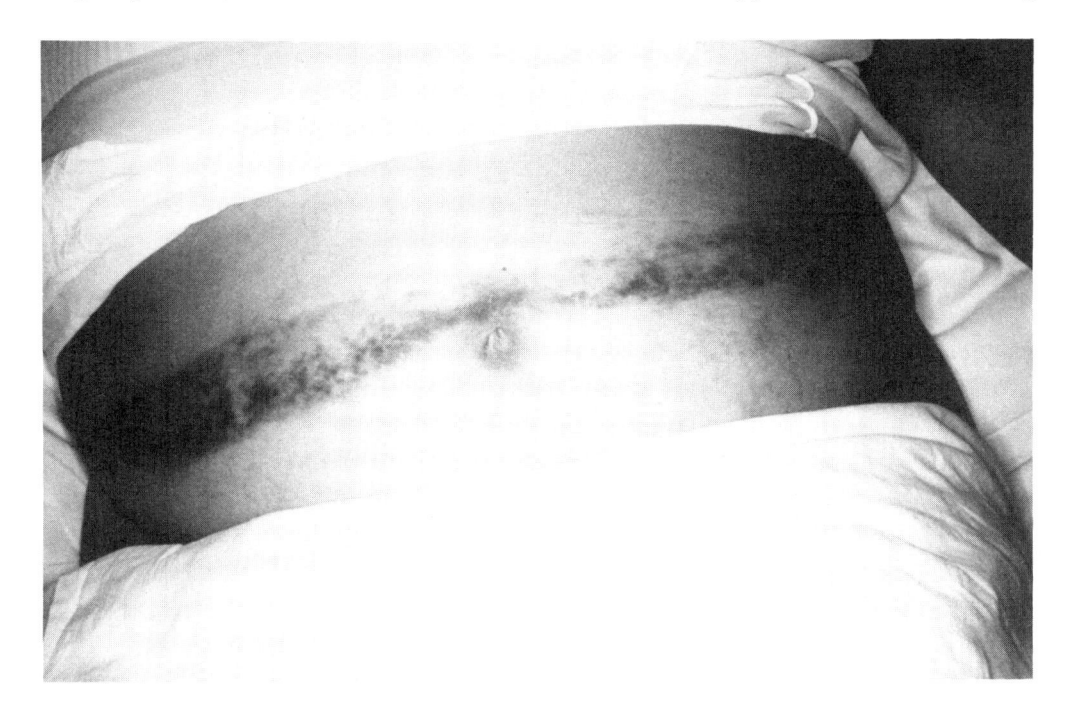

Figure 4.5

341. A likely injury she may have sustained would be

 (A) perforated colon
 (B) ruptured spleen
 (C) mesenteric vascular avulsion
 (D) fractured pelvis
 (E) pneumothorax

342. She obviously had a considerable deceleration force spread out over surface and time in what constitutes

 (A) penetrating trauma
 (B) torsion injury
 (C) blunt trauma
 (D) hypertension
 (E) vertical deceleration

343. Each of the following clinical indicators of intra-abdominal injury is useful **EXCEPT**:

   (A)   abdominal tenderness
   (B)   paracentesis
   (C)   CT scan
   (D)   peritoneal lavage
   (E)   arteriography

ANSWERS AND TUTORIAL ON ITEMS 341-343

The answers are: **341-B; 342-C; 343-A**.

This patient was obviously wearing her seat belt! The bruise around the abdomen from the mark of the seat belt shows that she sustained a considerable deceleration force, and at least as evident from the soft tissue of the abdomen superficially, this constituted a significant blunt trauma. In blunt trauma to the abdomen, some of the more sensitive tissues and organs may be disrupted, and a ruptured spleen would be the most likely visceral injury sustained from this vehicular blunt trauma. The other injuries listed are possible, but probably the spleen would rupture before any of the others attain a threshold clinical injury significance.

With respect to evaluation of such an abdominal injury, each of the invasive or radiographic studies may be helpful. However, one cannot follow abdominal tenderness in a patient who already has evidence of a significant abdominal wall injury. It is unlikely that her abdomen would be nontender even without any translation of this force into the viscera beneath this very large surface bruise from the secondary impact with a seat belt.

Items 344-346

One of the emergency room "regulars" is seen for a very distended and puffy hand and fever. His upper arm and forearm are seen in **Figure 4.6** at the time of examination.

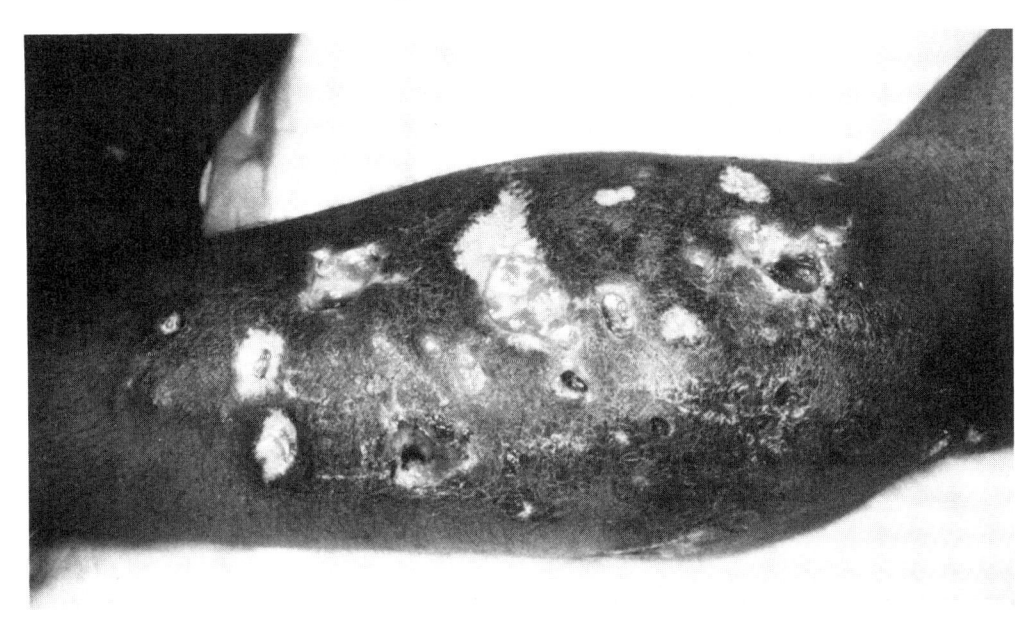

Figure 4.6

344. The underlying diagnosis is

    (A) chronic granulomatous disease
    (B) heroin addiction
    (C) mycosis fungoides
    (D) histoplasmosis
    (E) epidermoid carcinoma

345. One of the systemic complications of this condition is

    (A) tricuspid valvulitis
    (B) glomerulonephritis
    (C) urosepsis
    (D) hepatic metastasis
    (E) aplastic anemia

141

346. Each of the following is an actual complication of the condition portrayed **EXCEPT**:

   (A) osteomyelitis
   (B) digital gangrene
   (C) Volkmann's ischemic contracture
   (D) clostridial septicemia
   (E) carcinogenesis

ANSWERS AND TUTORIAL ON ITEMS 344-346

The answers are: **344-B; 345-A; 346-E**.

This patient is a "skin popper" injecting heroin and the excipient with which it is mixed under the subcutaneous tissue. This is often done in search for a vein, which veins are often obliterated early in the course of the addiction. For that reason, the patient then may seek out arterial injection sites, both for vascular access and also for the special sensation known as a "hand trip" or "flash" which may be partly due to the drug, but in a large part is due to catecholamine release and excipient embolization. Some of the excipients with which the heroin powder is mixed include quinine and talc. The former aids oxidation-reduction potential favoring anaerobic organisms and clostridial septicemia is a possibility. Because of the arterial embolization and ischemia, Volkmann's ischemic contracture is possible, as well as bone infections, osteomyelitis, and soft tissue destruction. Of all the complications reported, that include right heart valvulitis and migratory pulmonary emboli, carcinogenesis of the infected area is not likely amid all the other sequelae of drug abuse.

Items 347-349

A 28 year-old is brought to the emergency room after a high impact automobile collision in which he lost consciousness and broke several ribs. An aortogram (**Figure 4.7**) is obtained after widened mediastinum was suggested on chest X-ray.

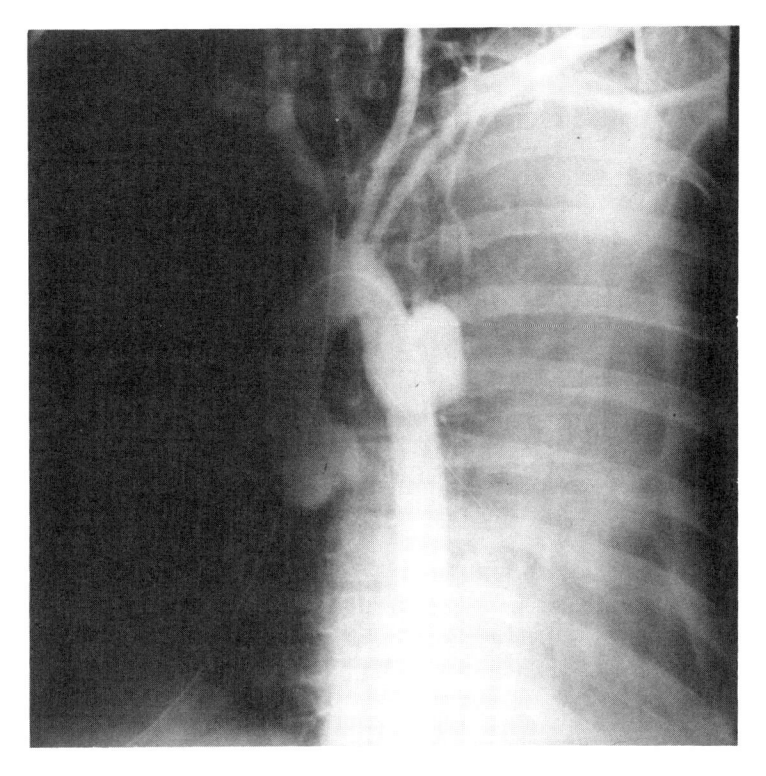

Figure 4.7

347. The X-ray shows

   (A) a luetic aneurysm
   (B) ruptured sinus of Valsalva
   (C) congenital patent ductus arteriosus
   (D) coarctation of the aorta
   (E) traumatic aortic arch aneurysm

348. The anatomic region of this defect is characteristic because

   (A) it is the center of frontal impact of the chest
   (B) the azygous vein crosses at this site
   (C) the *ligamentum arteriosum* tethers the aorta at this site
   (D) the pericardium is attenuated at this location
   (E) the aorta crosses the bony spine at this position

349. The demonstration of this lesion should be followed by

　　(A)　advice on avoiding hypertension
　　(B)　close check on renal function
　　(C)　analgesics for pain
　　(D)　vasodilators
　　(E)　thoracotomy

ANSWERS AND TUTORIAL ON ITEMS 347-349

The answers are: **347-E; 348-C; 349-E**.

　　This injury is a classic one from frontal deceleration of the "steering post collision" type. In this instance of rapid deceleration in the automobile accident, the heart literally "jumps off the aorta". The reason that this particular anatomic site is characteristically involved in this aortic disruption is that it is at this point that the *ligamentum arteriosum* tethers the aorta. When the heart and great vessels are thrown forward in the chest, it is at the site of this fixation that the tearing occurs, resulting in this aortic arch aneurysm.
　　Hypertension makes this lesion worse, and some control through the use of medication or otherwise would be necessary to be sure that the aortic arch aneurysm that is traumatic in origin does not dissect. However, thoracotomy is the method for treatment with a repair of this arch aneurysm probably by vascular prosthetic arch replacement.

Items 350-352

An African child was burned in a cooking fire and came for attention after the result seen in **Figure 4.8A** and **Figure 4.8B**. In the OR, the operation is shown in **Figure 4.8C**, with the postoperative result seen in **Figure 4.8D**.

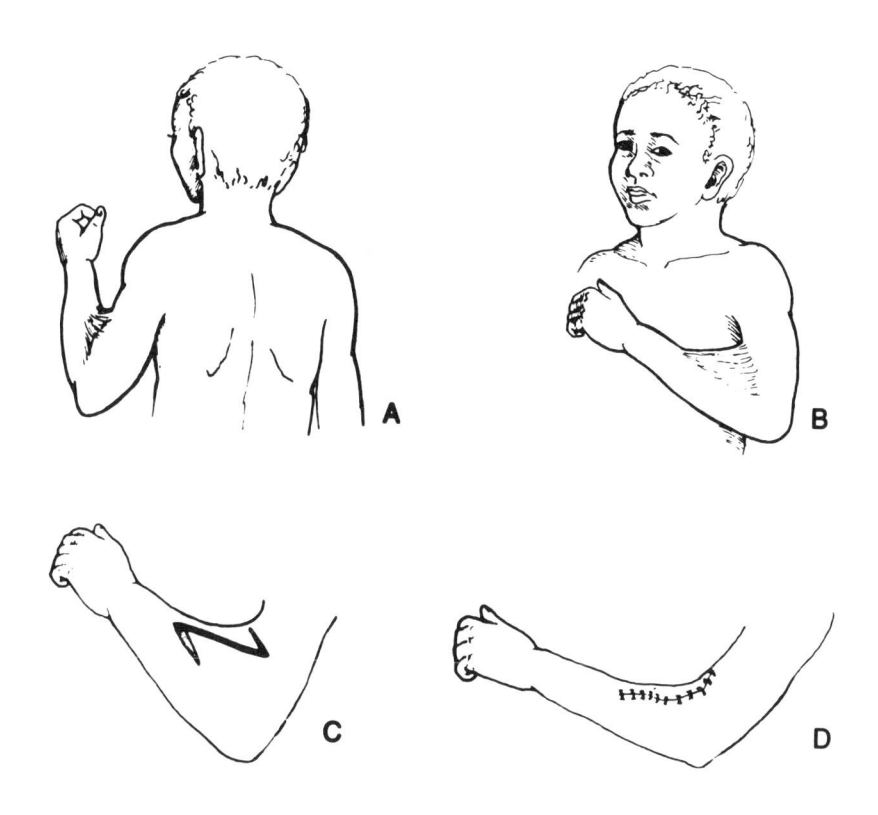

Figure 4.8

350. The operation performed was

   (A) split thickness skin grafts
   (B) microvascular composite grafts
   (C) Z-plasty incisions
   (D) tube pedicle graft
   (E) tendon transfer

351. The principle purpose of the procedure is

   (A) cosmetic rehabilitation
   (B) prevent fused joint
   (C) straighten vascular channels
   (D) release of scar contracture
   (E) improve sensation

352. The result is

   (A) a functional upper extremity
   (B) improved appearance
   (C) better range of shoulder motion
   (D) decreased pain
   (E) increased blood flow

ANSWERS AND TUTORIAL ON ITEMS 350-352

The answers are: **350-C; 351-D; 352-A.**

This child has the disability seen with joint contracture from burns that heal by scarring with a web causing immobilization of very valuable joints. In the lower extremity, such mobility can be sacrificed with less disability, but the burn contracture of the elbow leads to a useless upper extremity. Before this is allowed to persist for many years and not only cause considerable joint and other disuse atrophy in a child who would learn other compensations and accommodate this disability through never having attained skills in the use of this arm, rehabilitation by reconstruction is important.

The form that rehabilitation takes in this instance is Z-plasty scar contracture release. In this technique, an incision is made in the contracting web in the form of a "Z", and the triangular flaps interposed to disrupt the web contracture and to lengthen and make more useful the upper extremity that can be seen in extension postoperatively.

Items 353-362

353. A 28 year-old man enters the emergency room with sudden onset of severe abdominal pain radiating from left groin to the back and down to the scrotum. He has nausea and urinary frequency and is very restless, without ability to get comfortable in any position, although on physical examination he has no remarkable findings except for his agitation. He has had no previous illness. These findings are suggestive of

(A) sigmoid diverticulitis
(B) porphyria attack
(C) acute cholecystitis
(D) left ureteral calculus
(E) acute appendicitis

354. A 19 year-old woman is brought to the emergency room pale and listless with thready pulse. She has abdominal tenderness and cervical tenderness on pelvic examination which suggests a right pelvic mass. These findings are characteristic of

(A) ruptured appendicitis with abscess
(B) torsion of an ovarian cyst
(C) ruptured ectopic pregnancy
(D) strangulated internal hernia
(E) acute tubo-ovarian abscess

355. A 6 year-old boy is riding his bicycle when he develops a right scrotal pain that brings him crying to his mother. On examination the left side of the scrotum appears normal, but the right testicle appears retracted, tender, dusky, and does not transluminate with a flashlight. These findings are characteristic of

(A) torsion of the appendix testis
(B) torsion of the right testicle
(C) appendicitis
(D) strangulated right inguinal hernia
(E) expanding right hydrocele

356. A 29 year-old man is playing tennis and experiences an audible "snap" and pain just below the popliteal space where there is some discoloration in the area and tenderness. The patient is able to walk with some discomfort, and a small "knot" is palpable in the tender area of the upper calf. This is characteristic of

   (A) ruptured popliteal aneurysm
   (B) acute Baker's cyst
   (C) ruptured plantaris muscle
   (D) ruptured Achilles tendon
   (E) ruptured superficial varicose vein

357. A 40 year-old obese woman enters the emergency room with acute onset of upper abdominal pain 30 minutes after a lunch of fried foods. She denies alcohol intake, and any prior history of dyspepsia. The pain radiates through to her back and the abdominal tenderness is located just to the right side of the epigastric midline. The likely clinical scenario suggests

   (A) acute duodenal ulcer
   (B) acute cholecystitis
   (C) acute pancreatitis
   (D) myocardial infarction
   (E) reflux esophagitis

358. A 68 year-old smoker complains of acute onset of right leg pain and numbness with inability to walk since the event began suddenly two hours before. He had two previous myocardial infarctions and is on digitalis, which recently regularized atrial fibrillation for which he had been most recently treated. On examination the left leg is cold below mid-thigh, pale, and pulseless. This clinical pattern is compatible with

   (A) deep venous thrombosis
   (B) superficial thrombophlebitis
   (C) aortic-iliac atherosclerotic disease
   (D) femoral arterial embolism
   (E) angiosclerosis obliterans

359. A 16 year-old boy reports to the emergency room with abdominal pain of 12 hours duration that began in the periumbilical area and migrated to the right lower quadrant. Which of the following physical findings most strongly suggests acute appendicitis?

   (A) direct abdominal tenderness at McBurney's point
   (B) rebound tenderness referred to the umbilicus
   (C) a positive psoas sign
   (D) rectal examination tenderness
   (E) high-pitched tinkling bowel sounds

360. A 72 year-old man is brought to the emergency room after complaining of sudden onset of backache and abdominal pain with one episode of a loose bloody bowel movement. On physical examination, a poorly defined midline abdominal mass is palpable, and his blood pressure is low, although he has been under treatment for hypertension. A likely cause for these findings is

   (A)   obstructing carcinoma of the colon
   (B)   sigmoid volvulus
   (C)   expanding aortic aneurysm
   (D)   ischemic colitis
   (E)   mesenteric infarction

361. A 68 year-old woman is brought by her daughter who has found her mumbling incoherently three days after a similar episode in which she was unable to see clearly all of any object placed before her. A transient period of forgetfulness resolved but now similar impairments appear to have returned. The likely diagnosis is

   (A)   amaurosis fujax
   (B)   toxic amblyopia
   (C)   retinal arteritis
   (D)   expanding intracranial aneurysm
   (E)   occlusive carotid artery stenosis

362. A 40 year-old woman is rushed to the emergency room following an automobile accident in which the she was slammed into the steering wheel and post. The patient has a large bruise across the anterior chest and has a bluish coloration of the face with distended neck veins. Stethoscope reveals barely audible heart sounds. The likely diagnosis is

   (A)   tension pneumothorax
   (B)   traumatic thoracic aortic aneurysm
   (C)   acute mediastinitis
   (D)   flail chest
   (E)   acute pericardial tamponade

ANSWERS AND TUTORIALS ON ITEMS 353-362

The answers are: **353-D; 354-C; 355-B; 356-C; 357-B; 358-D; 359-A; 360-C; 361-A; 362-E**.

353. The passage of a kidney stone in a previously healthy young man is typically characterized by acute flank and groin pain radiating to the scrotum. The other intra-abdominal crises should be manifest by peritoneal signs, and the patient would be typically protecting inflamed peritoneum by trying to minimize motion. Although always a possibility, appendicitis is less likely to give the kind and distribution of acute pain of sudden onset as described, and would likely show further physical findings.

354. The combination of abdominal pain, mass, and shock would suggest hemorrhage from some intra-abdominal catastrophe. Appendicitis and tubo-ovarian abscess are both possible in this age group, but would typically give inflammatory peritoneal symptoms before the abrupt onset of shock. A cyst or internal hernia is possible, but less probable than a tubal pregnancy, the rupture of which results in far more blood loss more quickly. Pregnancy is assumed for any woman of reproductive age, until it is ruled out, and in this instance is the most likely cause of the acute abdominal catastrophe described.

355. Torsion of the appendix testis may give pain and does cause an elevation and tenderness in the testis in the early stages, but it transluminates as a black dot in the scrotum. Hernia and hydrocele would give more presentation in the groin and less evidence of scrotal discomfort; whereas, appendicitis would give abdominal peritoneal findings. Torsion of the testis often presents following some evidence of physical exertion as in the setting described.

356. The patient would be unable to stand let alone walk if it had been the Achilles tendon that ruptured, and the other acute events in the popliteal space are not common in this setting. Although varicose veins may occasionally leak subcutaneously, the acute setting here and the context of the event suggest rupture of the plantaris muscle. It is annoying, but not disabling.

357. The relationship of the onset of pain to meals is frequently helpful for the upper gastrointestinal tract, since peptic ulcer is most significant at times of unopposed acid secretion, therefore is often relieved by eating. Fatty food intolerance is associated with biliary tract disease, and it in turn may lead to pancreatitis. However, the pain of pancreatitis is often more severe, and is not as localized to the right of the epigastrium. Both myocardial and esophageal symptoms do not typically localize to the abdomen radiating to the back, and usually have some prior signals of antecedent disease.

358. Myocardial infarction can give rise to mural thrombus which may remain in the heart during fibrillation, but with improved contractility and regularization of the ventricular output, thromboembolism may result. The most likely point for impact is in the narrowing of the femoral artery at the adductor canal, giving rise to a threatened limb from distal arterial occlusion. Atherosclerosis and other gradually progressive vascular disorders may also result in ischemia, but are less likely to be as abrupt in onset. Both superficial and deep venous thrombosis can compromise circulation, but on the venous side of the circulation there would be an additional threat of pulmonary thromboembolism from the deep venous system, not made more likely by regularized myocardial rhythm.

359. Direct abdominal tenderness at the site of the appendix is the most suggestive physical finding for the diagnosis of appendicitis at the early stage when the appendix alone is inflamed. Rebound tenderness may detect peritoneal signs when the parietal peritoneum is involved, and psoas and rectal lateralizaton may be helpful for retroperitoneal findings but less frequently. Point tenderness remains a *sine qua non* as an operative indication for acute appendicitis.

360. Abdominal aneurysm is a likelihood in a patient who presents with a midline mass, particularly if pulsating laterally, and the symptoms and evidence of acute bowel ischemia suggest that it is rupturing and occluding visceral branches, as does hypotension. This constitutes a vascular emergency and is life threatening. Colon carcinoma and sigmoid volvulus might give blood loss, but not typically abdominal pain that begins as back pain but progresses rapidly.

361. Transient focal ischemic attacks, particularly involving visual field abnormalities that come and go, are often associated with thromboembolic cerebral circulation impairment. A frequent cause of this is an ulcerated arterial sclerotic plaque which gives rise to platelet aggregates and microthrombi that break loose from the atherosclerotic endothelial ulcerated surface. This finding is an indication for carotid artery flow and imaging studies and correction as indicated.

362. Deceleration injury can result in hemopericardium, either from bleeding into the pericardial space from vessels around the heart or from rupture of one of the heart's chambers. If this blood accumulates under systolic arterial pressure, decompensation is rapid, since outflow will cease, although it takes a longer time for compromise if the pressure is that of the right ventricle or diastolic or systemic venous pressure. Tension pneumothorax can also cause distended neck veins, but would not change heart sounds. A thoracic aneurysm could rupture into the pericardium, but then the acute effect of it would be the same as pericardial tamponade. Acute mediastinitis would not develop this rapidly following injury whether from esophageal perforation or other origin.

Items 363-372

363. Post-traumatic pulmonary insufficiency ("shock lung") with onset suggested in the 24 hours following injury is likely **NOT** to involve incrimination of which of the following insults?

    (A) oxygen toxicity
    (B) pulmonary fat embolism
    (C) toxic gas inhalation
    (D) perfusion with enzymes from pancreatic injury
    (E) microaggregated debris from bank blood

364. Which of the following perfusion beds in shock has the greatest ability to regulate its blood flow and the greatest adaptation to decreased perfusion pressure?

    (A) liver
    (B) brain
    (C) lung
    (D) heart
    (E) kidney

365. Each of the following treatments has been used in the management of fat embolism, until our information on the syndrome has been improved, so that which is now contraindicated?

    (A) controlled increased oxygen tension ventilation
    (B) positive end expiratory pressure
    (C) heparin therapy
    (D) stabilization of long bone fractures
    (E) high frequency "jet" ventilation

366. The most clinically significant early physiologic abnormality in post-traumatic pulmonary insufficiency is

    (A) increased physiologic shunt
    (B) increased dead space
    (C) ventilator barotrauma
    (D) cardiogenic pulmonary edema
    (E) pulmonary fibrosis

367. Which of the following statements is true concerning transfusion with banked whole blood?

   (A) it has a hematocrit equal to that of the donor at the time of the blood donation
   (B) it contains sufficient numbers of active platelets for hemostasis purposes
   (C) it is the treatment of choice for anemic patients with respiratory complications
   (D) it is hyperkalemic
   (E) it is alkaline

368. Advantages of crystalloid solution over colloid in fluid resuscitation include all of the following **EXCEPT**:

   (A) cost
   (B) availability
   (C) retrievability
   (D) low pyrogenicity
   (E) edema

369. Military Anti-Shock Trousers (MAST trousers) should be removed from the patient

   (A) on arrival in the emergency room
   (B) in order to allow the patient to empty the bladder
   (C) in the operating room following fluid resuscitation
   (D) only after lower extremity and pelvic fractures are stabilized
   (E) as soon as possible to facilitate extremity neurologic and vascular examination

370. Which of these patients is **LEAST** likely to be in shock? A patient

   (A) making a normal quantity of normal quality urine
   (B) with a normal blood pressure
   (C) with a cardiac output three times normal
   (D) whose extremities are warm and pink
   (E) with hypotension and severe bradycardia

371. Caloric energy requirements in patients with a high metabolic demand, such as a major body surface thermal burn or comparable internal surface chemical burn as from peritonitis from perforated ulcer, may require daily caloric intake for the average size adult of

   (A) 500 kcal
   (B) 1000 kcal
   (C) 2000 kcal
   (D) 2500 kcal
   (E) 3000 kcal

372. Which of the following vital signs most closely represents a patient with closed head trauma that results in loss of consciousness?

(A) increased pulse, increased blood pressure
(B) decreased pulse, increased blood pressure
(C) increased pulse, decreased blood pressure
(D) decreased pulse, decreased blood pressure
(E) normal pulse, normal blood pressure

ANSWERS AND TUTORIALS ON ITEMS 363-372

The answers are: **363-A; 364-E; 365-C; 366-A; 367-D; 368-E; 369-C; 370-A; 371-E; 372-B.**

363. Oxygen toxicity and barotrauma from ventilator therapy are possible complications leading to pulmonary injury following trauma, but not within the first 24 hours. In this event, more direct injury from the inhalation route from toxic gas or from the perfusion side, such as with lytic enzymes or microaggregated debris from bank blood or long bone fracture giving rise to fat embolism, are more likely culprits.

364. Over a wide range of perfusion pressures, the kidney has amazing adaptive responses to adjust its perfusion. First, it autoregulates its resistance vessels so that they relax with decreased perfusion pressure which tends to maintain constant flow. However, when mean arterial pressure is below 80 mm Hg, the kidneys release renin, which results in the pressor activity of angiotensin II, thereby increasing perfusion pressure through peripheral vasoconstriction. A third step is taken by the same angiotensin II in stimulating the outer layer of the adrenal cortex to release the mineralocorticoid aldosterone which ultimately results in sodium retention and volume expansion. These built-in adaptations allow the kidney resiliency in hypoperfusion not shared by such organs with a marginal arterial supply such as the liver with few adaptive responses. The internal vascular resistance of the brain is largely regulated by partial gas tensions (particularly P_{CO_2}), but are quickly used up in adaptive response. Each of the other visceral organs listed does not have the reserves and protective mechanisms of the kidney, and suffer dysfunction earlier in shock.

365. Careful support of respiration by enriched, but not toxic, levels of oxygen and increased end expiratory pressures but short of barotrauma to the lung, (for which jet ventilation may be useful), are measures that support the patient with respiratory distress. Decreasing further fat embolization may take place with early fixation of fractures, by open reduction if necessary. Heparin has lipolytic activity. It was formerly given for this effect, but thereby converted free fat globules to the more toxic free fatty acids, which actually exacerbated pulmonary injury, so that heparin is now contraindicated.

366. Shock lung has increased fluid content, much of it interstitial. This increased fluid volume and decreased gas space has lead to a greater fraction of the lung perfused but not ventilated which is by definition the physiologic shunt. Pulmonary fibrosis occurs at a very late stage and can inhibit gas exchange and impair compliance. This same alveolar capillary blockade can occur from lung injury by high pressures or oxygen tensions administered to the lung. However, the physiologic basis for the inability of the lung to oxygenate blood adequately is the greater fraction of lung perfused without effective ventilation, that is, physiologic shunt.

367. Dr. F.D. Moore described the "ancient and honorable whole blood transfusion" as: "cold, acidotic (sic), hyperkalemic, thrombocytopenic" and without any functioning white cells with only respiratory function in the decaying residual erythrocyte mass. It is not the treatment of choice for anemia. In fact, there are very rare indications for whole blood transfusion and not many of those would involve prolonged storage. For most other purposes of expanding oxygen transport capacity, red blood cells would be more appropriate and for volume expansion crystalloid or colloid would be preferable to whole blood. Donated blood is diluted in the anticoagulant to wind up with a hematocrit lower than that of the donor, and the preservatives are acidic solutions, while potassium increases in concentration as it leeches from devitalized cells.

368. Crystalloid solution is readily available at 1/20th of the cost of albumin, and has fewer associated pyrogenic reactions. It is also possible to retrieve infused crystalloid through diuresis in patients with functioning kidneys. It does cross permeable membranes to accumulate in "third space" components of extracellular fluid; whereas, albumin has a longer circulating half life in patients tending toward congestive edema.

369. Whenever "autotransfusion" results from application of MAST trousers and increased peripheral resistance to prevent pooling in the lower extremities, this same accomplished reinfusion could work against the patient if the MAST trousers were removed prematurely before fluid resuscitation. This should not be carried out in the emergency room to facilitate examination, to return the trousers to the ambulance crew or before adequate resuscitation. MAST trousers are not appropriate as stabilization of fractures. The compressive effect on the urinary bladder from intra-abdominal increase in pressure occurs as soon as the trousers are put on, and voiding or catheterization should occur while they are in place. Hypotension and a reversal of the fluid sequestration from the circulation occurs in premature removal until definitive surgical control can be achieved with adequate volume resuscitation.

370. The kidney is a vital perfusion bed that reflects its blood flow by autoregulating its resistance and endocrine actions that result in pressor activity and volume expansion. Only after these protective mechanisms are exhausted and hypoperfusion occurs does the quality and quantity of urine decrease, so a patient making normal urine is not in shock. In contrast, a patient with a normal blood pressure may have elevated this pressure from hypotensive levels by endogenous or administered catecholamines or other increased resistance. A patient with a higher cardiac output or warm and suffused extremities may be in endotoxic shock. The patient who has intra-abdominal hemorrhage as well as a closed head injury may have hypotension and the Cushing reflex leading to bradycardia from elevated intracranial pressure. Blood pressure and evidence of extremity blood flow are less reliable than the function of one vital visceral perfusion bed that has an output to reflect its perfusion, and the other examples listed would have impaired urine output or concentration.

371. Burn patients experience very high calorie requirements that may be 25 kcal/kg body weight plus 40 kcal per percent of body surface burned.

372. Closed head injury may result in the Cushing reflex which is a reflection of increased intracranial pressure. This gives rise to a strong vagal discharge, and that is reflected in a bradycardia which slows pulse and increased resistance which raises the blood pressure. If a patient has hypotension with a closed head injury, the source of the hypotension must be found in probable blood loss somewhere other than in the head, with the rare exception being in newborns or infants.

Cushing reflex: ↓HR, ↑BP

CHAPTER V
HEAD AND NECK SURGERY
ENDOCRINE SURGERY

Items 373-375

This 12 year-old boy had noted a neck lump for most of his life, recently enlarging. Exploration in the OR reveals the specimen shown in **Figure 5.1**.

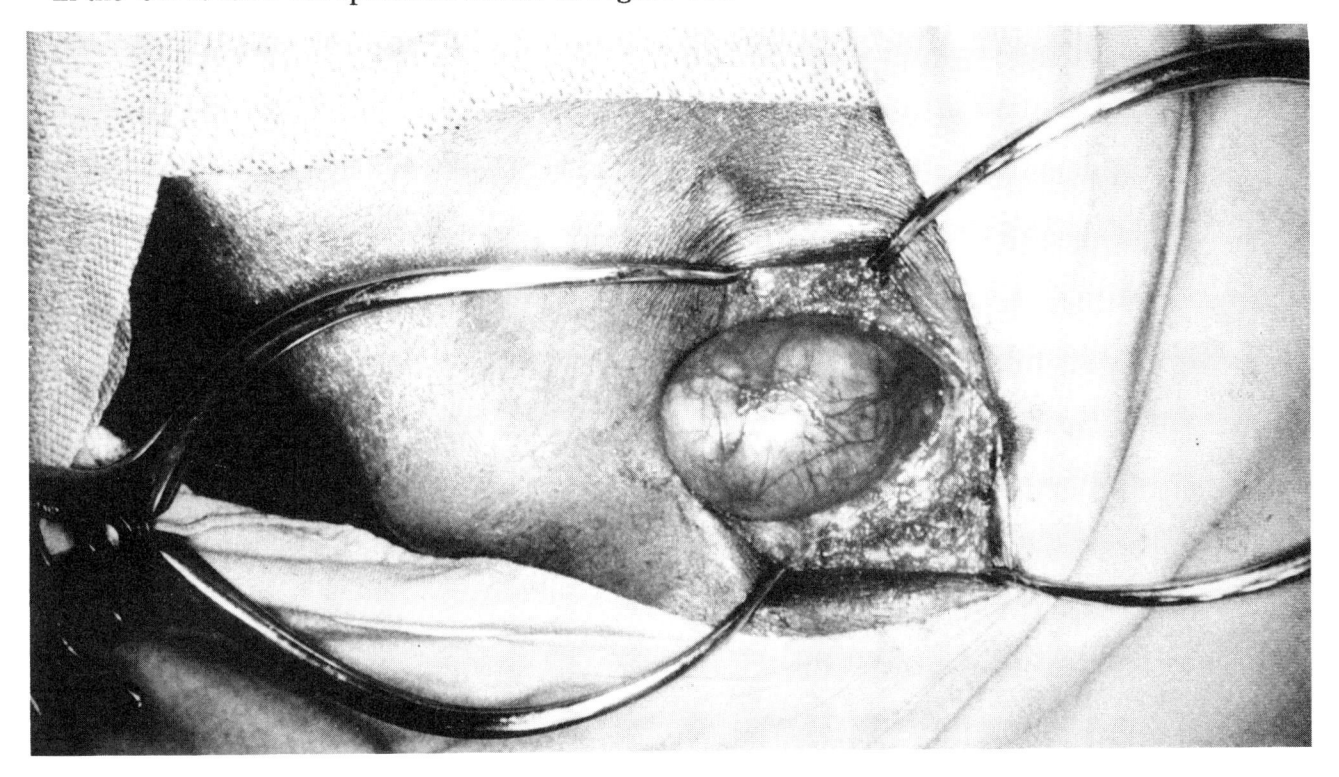

Figure 5.1

373. It is a derivative of the

    (A)   thyroglossal tract
    (B)   neuroectoderm
    (C)   first pharyngeal pouch
    (D)   second pharyngeal pouch
    (E)   dental anlage

374. On cut section it would be

   (A) a solid tumor
   (B) a pseudocyst
   (C) hemorrhagic
   (D) filled with colloid
   (E) containing cystic secretions

375. The most likely complication would be

   (A) malignant degeneration
   (B) infection
   (C) fistula formation
   (D) hypothyroidism
   (E) sialolithiasis

ANSWERS AND TUTORIAL ON ITEMS 373-375

The answers are: **373-D; 374-E; 375-B**.

This clinical photograph is of a second pharyngeal pouch cyst presenting in the classic position. The first pharyngeal pouch is at the level of the external auditory meatus. The boy has had it most of his life, and the "rule of sevens" suggests that this is likely to be congenital (seven days inflammatory, seven months neoplastic and seven years congenital). This one, in fact, was filled with cystic secretion materials with a sebaceous character; many can be purulent when secondarily infected. That secondary infection is the most likely complication, and if there is interior communication and incision and drainage is done, fistula formation may result, but that is less common than infection which is the usual complicating feature to which it is predisposed.

Items 376-378

The lesion shown in **Figure 5.2** has been making the patient aware of an odd taste for five months and in the last two months has interfered with speech.

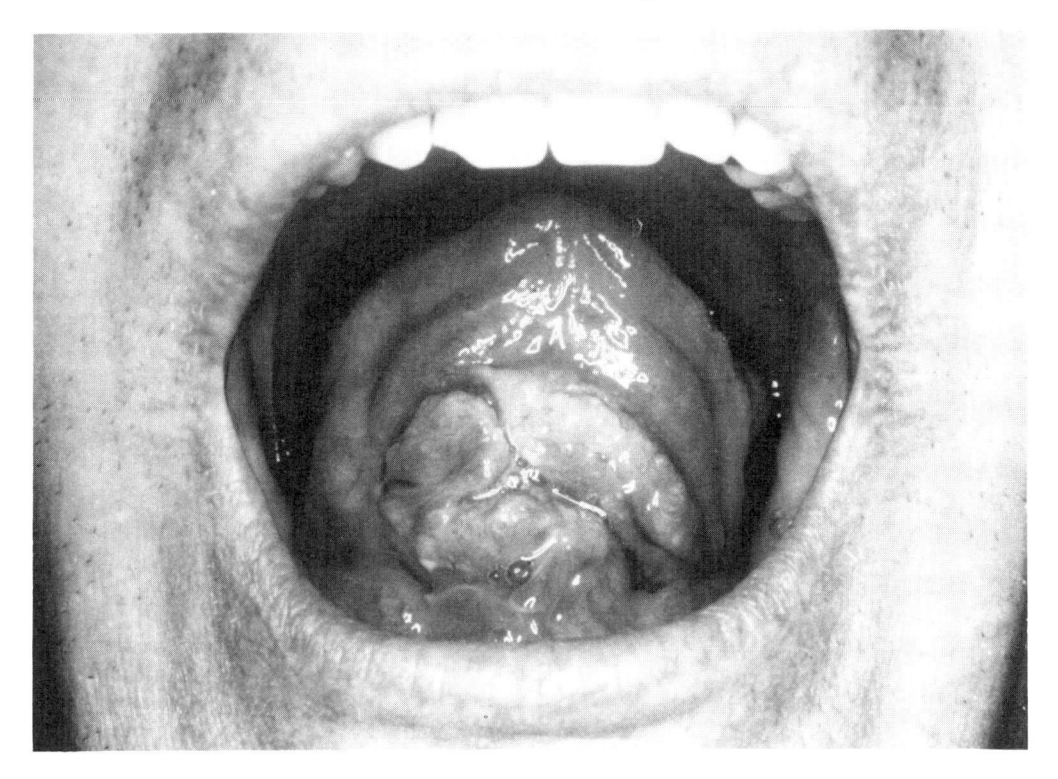

Figure 5.2

376. It is most probably

 (A) congenital
 (B) inflammatory
 (C) benign
 (D) malignant
 (E) secretory

377. The histopathologic examination after biopsy would show

 (A) adenocarcinoma
 (B) squamous cell carcinoma
 (C) leiomyosarcoma
 (D) lipoma
 (E) secretory cysts

159

378. Treatment will be limited to

   (A) radiotherapy
   (B) local excision
   (C) incisional biopsy
   (D) commando composite resection with radical neck dissection
   (E) skin graft to anterior undersurface of the tongue

ANSWERS AND TUTORIAL ON ITEMS 376-378

The answers are: **376-D; 377-B; 378-D**.

There are some benign lesions that exist under the anterior surface of the tongue and adjacent structures such as ranula and epulis, and this is not one of them. This is an ulcerated form of squamous cell carcinoma proven by a small incisional biopsy in the planning for the several stage treatment that will involve a very extensive operation in order to get control of the margins and resurface the floor of the mouth following the neck dissection.

Items 379-381

A 60 year-old woman had a painless mass appear at the right angle of the jaw. The appearance of the mass (**Figure 5.3A**) is confirmed by operative exploration (**Figure 5.3B**).

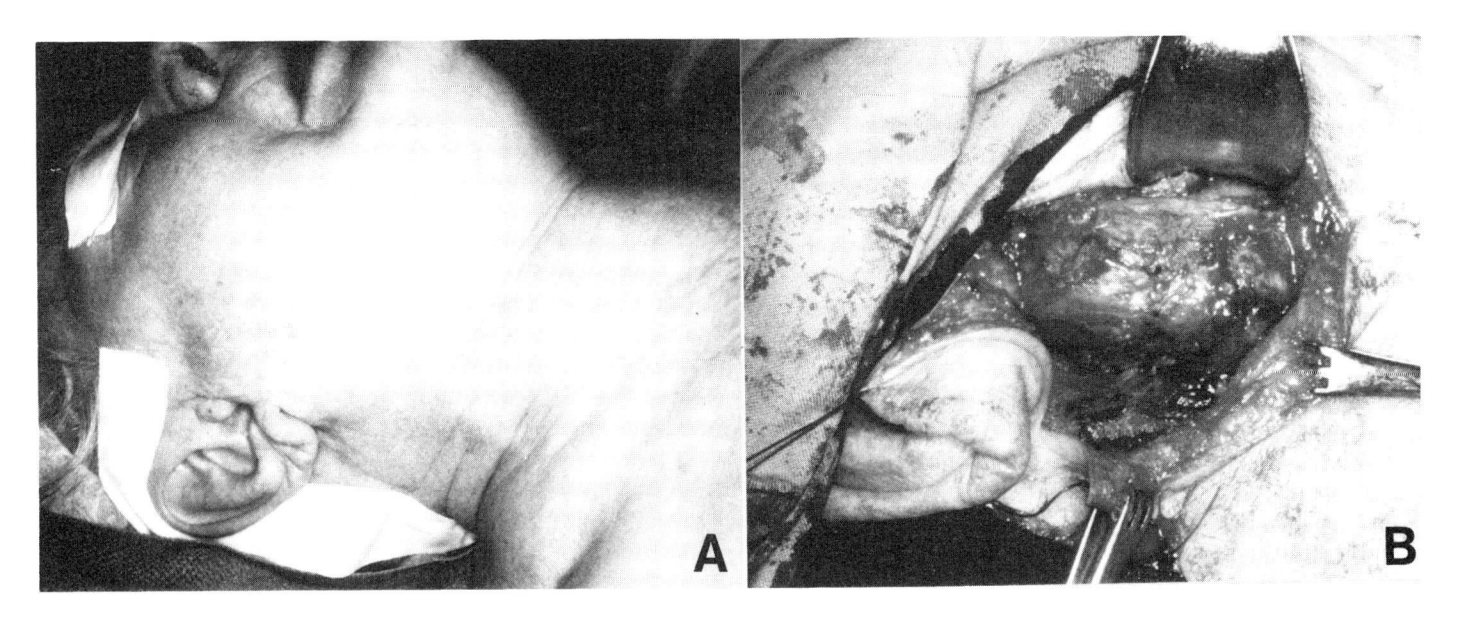

Figure 5.3

379. The finding is

   (A) vascular in origin
   (B) neural derivative
   (C) superficial glandular
   (D) deep glandular
   (E) lymphatic

380. The probable histology of the mass is

   (A) benign neoplasm
   (B) inflammatory
   (C) malignant neoplasm
   (D) hematologic
   (E) nerve sheath

381. Treatment should be by

    (A)   radiotherapy
    (B)   superficial gland resection
    (C)   chemotherapy
    (D)   radical composite resection
    (E)   biopsy only

ANSWERS AND TUTORIAL ON ITEMS 379-381

The answers are: **379-C; 380-A; 381-B**.

This patient has the clinical appearance of a superficial parotid tumor, confirmed at operative exploration. The most likely histology of the mass is that of a benign neoplasm. Because of the benign nature of the neoplasm, although it might tend toward local recurrence if not completely excised, superficial gland resection is the treatment carried out. There is no need for radical surgical resection and sacrifice of the facial nerve nor adjunctive chemo- or radiotherapy, but the mass should also not be ignored or biopsied only. Complete excision by superficial parotidectomy is followed by a highly successful control rate.

Items 382-385

(A) Adrenal cortical adenoma → Rx unilateral adrenalectomy
(B) Bilateral adrenocortical hyperplasia
(C) Both
(D) Neither

382. treated by subtotal bilateral adrenalectomy

383. invariably due to primary drive outside the adrenal

384. hypertension

385. malignant hypertension

ANSWERS AND TUTORIAL ON ITEMS 382-385

The answers are: **382-D; 383-D; 384-C; 385-D**.

Adrenal cortical adenoma can give rise to primary aldosteronism, Cushing's syndrome, and — much more rarely due to a benign adenoma — virilizing or masculinizing syndromes, depending on the principle cell type in which the adenoma arose: zona glomerulosa, fasciculata, and reticularis respectively. The same features, however, can be produced by the same secretions based not in a benign adenoma but bilateral (micronodular) hyperplasia. In the instance of Cushing's disease, this hyperplasia is due to the stimulation of ACTH from pituitary or ectopic para-endocrine source of peptide secretion. Therefore for Cushing's syndrome, adrenocortical hyperplasia is secondary and only extremely rarely has hyperplasia been a primary autonomous adrenal source of Cushing's syndrome.

This is *not* the case for aldosteronism. In secondary aldosteronism there is an excess secretion from both adrenals secondary to renin and angiotensin driven stimulation, but there is also a not infrequent syndrome of primary aldosteronism based in bilateral micronodular cortical hyperplasia. In this case, this hyperplasia is not invariably due to a primary drive outside the adrenal gland, since this aldosteronism is primary.

Whether due to an outside peptide stimulus or due to a primary autonomous hyperfunction, bilateral cortical hyperplasia should *not* be treated by subtotal bilateral adrenalectomy. The reason for this is that it will inevitably recur whether or not it is responding to an external drive. Bilateral micronodular hyperplasia in primary aldosteronism is not successfully treated by bilateral subtotal adrenalectomy. In addition, bilateral total adrenalectomy carries the very high disadvantage of requiring corticosteroid replacement therapy, a price too high to pay for a disease that can be managed by medication that is less dangerous with a higher margin of safety. Both primary aldosteronism and Cushing's syndrome have associated hypertension. In neither case is this hypertension a malignant hypertension, and each is relatively easily managed without desperate complications based in hypertension.

Items 386-389

        (A)   Parotid gland tumor
        (B)   Submandibular gland tumor
        (C)   Both
        (D)   Neither

386. sialolithiasis

387. 80% benign

388. high recurrence rate

389. "commando" composite resection

ANSWERS AND TUTORIAL ON ITEMS 386-389

The answers are: **386-C; 387-A; 388-C; 389-B**.

Parotid gland tumors are usually benign, may grow huge, and are resectable for cure, but with a high recurrence rate. Submandibular gland tumors are almost always malignant, have a high recurrence rate, and require extensive composite surgical resection such as the "commando" mandibulectomy/floor of the mouth excision with radical neck dissection. Both of the salivary glands may have ductal stones, but these are more frequently associated with inflammatory conditions than malignant ones. Calcification may be seen on X-ray that may be part of the sialolithiasis, inflammatory salivary gland changes or benign or malignant tumors in each location.

Items 390-393

        (A)   Papillary thyroid cancer
        (B)   Follicular thyroid cancer
        (C)   Both
        (D)   Neither

390.   increasing incidence

391.   high cure rate

392.   hematogenous spread

393.   external beam radiation therapy

ANSWERS AND TUTORIAL ON ITEMS 390-393

The answers are: **390-A; 391-C; 392-B; 393-D**.

    At the same time follicular thyroid cancer is decreasing in incidence as iodine deficiency and associated problems linked to it decrease, papillary thyroid carcinoma is increasing. Both tumors, however, have a high cure rate experienced with primary surgical therapy, particularly when adjunctive radioiodine therapy is added in follow-up for clinically significant thyroid cancer. This term refers to a presumed higher potential for malignant behavior, largely based on the patient's age, gender, tumor size and degree of differentiation.

    Follicular carcinoma does not primarily spread by means of lymphatic metastases, but hematogenous spread is most common for follicular thyroid cancer. This is not the case for papillary thyroid cancer. For neither of them is external beam radiation therapy a part of primary treatment. In selective instances of bony metastases for which thyroid cancer has a predilection, radiotherapy can be attempted, but only after a much more rational targeted source of ionizing radiation, i.e., radioiodine which can be taken up in the thyroid cells, particularly when enhanced with TSH by external administration or endogenous elevation from hypothyroidism that follows withholding thyroid replacement for a period of weeks.

Items 394-398

 (A) Repeat serum calcium
 (B) Urinary calcium
 (C) Serum parathormone
 (D) Thallium-technetium substraction scan
 (E) Ultrasound
 (F) Thyroid scan
 (G) Arteriogram
 (H) Venous sampling
 (I) CT scan
 (J) Surgical exploration

394. Next step for asymptomatic patient with diagnosed primary hyperparathyroidism with serum calcium 12.5 mg/dl.

395. Next step in hypercalcemic patient with unsuccessful parathyroid operation whose brother is now reported to have had the same result from the procedure.

396. A preferred procedure for a patient with suspected mediastinal parathyroid tumor who would like to avoid re-operation.

397. A study which can lateralize hypersecretion in the absence of an imaged mass.

398. A patient has had two calcium determinations one of 11.0 which caused a look back to records 3 years ago when it was 10.0. The next step should be

ANSWERS AND TUTORIAL ON ITEMS 394-398

The answers are: **394-J; 395-B; 396-G; 397-H; 398-A.**

 The patient with the established diagnosis of primary hyperparathyroidism requires no more localization than to locate an experienced parathyroid surgeon! The next step is surgical exploration, since it is this study that is both the most sensitive diagnostic localizing test as well as therapeutic in the vast majority of instances.
 In contrast, the patient who has had a failed primary cervical exploration and then only in retrospect is it found that a close relative has the same process, before localization studies should have a recheck of the primary diagnosis. Since the patient is documented hypercalcemic, a urinary calcium determination would be an appropriate test to determine whether there was a familial component based in hypocalciuria. The other possibility is that the patient is part of an endocrinologic kindred, and multiple endocrine adenopathy hyperparathyroidism is always based

in multiple gland disease. The most common source of failure in primary cervical operations that do not correct primary hyperparathyroidism is the failure to appreciate multiple gland disease and to correct it. If a patient has had a prior failed operation that does not find the focal source of the hyperparathyroidism and it is suspected in the mediastinum, if that mediastinal tumor is from the inferior thyroid arterial supply, a re-operation that is limited to the cervical approach can tease it back up into the cervicotomy incision along with the thymic extension. However, if the arterial supply is from the internal mammary artery, internal mammary arteriography can be carried out with staining of the tumor with hyperosmotic contrast material. This osmotic shock has destroyed the hyperfunction of parathyroid adenoma and has maintained successful control of hyperparathyroidism when followed for many years thereafter. This percutaneous procedure is an attractive alternative to sternotomy and those patients in whom that operation would otherwise be indicated.

An invasive lateralizing procedure that is helpful since it correlates form and function is venous sampling. That can be true even in the absence of an imaged mass. For example, if CT or arteriography had shown no evidence of a suspicious lesion in a postoperative patient's neck, venous sampling might be able to lateralize an elevated N-terminal parathormone secretion step-up on one side or the other of the neck, and exploration could begin with the site of the elevated parathormone.

A patient who has had an evident hypercalcemia requires that this be confirmed and that it is shown to be based in primary hyperparathyroidism. With respect to the one patient who is asymptomatic but had a calcium of 12.5 mg%, there is very little likelihood that he would remain asymptomatic for a prolonged period of time, and this operation should be restorative in sparing tissue that might suffer metastatic calcification as well as bone demineralization. In the patient with a calcium of 11 mg%, the course of such an asymptomatic patient might be observed if that were the preference, but first the diagnosis has to be confirmed. If the prior serum calcium was 10, and that (with the appropriate correction for albumin and judged against phosphate) is normal, the appropriate next step would be to repeat the serum calcium. If there were a steady trend upward, and the hypercalcemia on this occasion was proven not to be a fluke of random variation, then further determination could be made based in the other information from the SMA-12 determination (phosphate, chloride and albumin) and a parathormone ordered if appropriate based on these data.

Items 399-408

399. A mass in the midline of the neck just above the tracheal cartilage has been notable for some months in an 8 year-old girl but in the last four days there has been some reddening and discomfort. Which of the following statements is most likely to be correct?

   (A) it has a high probability of malignancy
   (B) it would most likely resolve completely with antibiotics
   (C) it would rise higher in the neck when she protrudes her tongue
   (D) incision and drainage is adequate treatment
   (E) it is associated with anomalies of the ear

400. Each of the following factors contributes to the likelihood that a mass in the neck is malignant **EXCEPT**:

   (A) the patient is alcoholic
   (B) the patient had another malignancy outside the neck
   (C) the patient is quite sure it was not present a week ago
   (D) the patient was a heavy smoker, but quit two years ago
   (E) the patient had facial irradiation for treatment of acne

401. A 19 year-old man is thrown forward in an automobile accident, striking his face on the dashboard. In the ER, his face was bloody and swollen with edematous tongue and a free floating mandible with multiple fractures of each ramus. There is an unresolved question of posterior cervical pain. Emergency management should include

   (A) nasotracheal intubation
   (B) emergency tracheotomy
   (C) cricothyroidotomy
   (D) oxygen by nasal catheter
   (E) splinting the neck in extension

402. Each of the following treatments is appropriate for Stage I carcinoma of the larynx **EXCEPT**:

   (A) laryngoscopic laser excision
   (B) primary radiotherapy
   (C) total laryngectomy
   (D) partial surgical excision
   (E) larynx-conserving subtotal hemilaryngectomy

403. Which of the following statements concerning parotid tumors is true?

    (A) 80% are benign
    (B) diagnosis is by incisional biopsy
    (C) facial nerve palsy is a definite sign of malignancy
    (D) tumors that extend into the deep lobe of the parotid are unresectable
    (E) radiation is an appropriate curative treatment

404. Which of the following statements is **NOT** true of vocal nodules?

    (A) they are a malignant tumor of the larynx
    (B) they are associated with chronic voice abuse as in screaming
    (C) they are sometimes called "singer's nodules"
    (D) they do regress with speech therapy
    (E) they are bilateral and located between anterior middle thirds of both true vocal cords

405. A debilitated patient in the inner city who has a problem with chronic alcoholism presents with weight loss, posterior cervical nodularity with ulceration, and leakage of a watery fluid that persisted in drainage for several months following outpatient incisional biopsy of neck nodes without any evidence of cancer. This clinical picture may represent a form of

    (A) bronchogenic cleft fistula
    (B) tuberculosis
    (C) squamous cell carcinoma
    (D) thyroid carcinoma
    (E) radiation necrosis

406. A 2 year-old child has been diagnosed with a capillary hemangioma which was noted shortly after birth and got larger along the left nasal margin between eye and lip for several months after it was first detected. It appears now to be regressing as the child grows, but the parents are asking if it can be treated before the child becomes self-conscious about its presence. Appropriate advice would be

    (A) to excise it with rotational full thickness skin-flap coverage
    (B) irradiation
    (C) surgical tattooing
    (D) embolization
    (E) temporizing

407. Each of the following is an indication for tonsillectomy **EXCEPT**:

 (A) dysphagia — interference with swallowing
 (B) dyspnea — interference with breathing from mass effect in the nasopharynx
 (C) peritonsillar abscess
 (D) bacterial allergy from focal infection
 (E) a second acute tonsillitis episode in a 4 year-old whose older brother is also scheduled for tonsillectomy

408. Following commando composite resection (mandibulectomy and anterior glossectomy for floor of the mouth squamous cell carcinoma), combined with bilateral radical neck dissection, a patient is seen in follow-up nine months postoperation. On examination you find three firm nontender nodules vertically aligned and spaced along the posterior cervical triangle, on the right, and — to your surprise — similar nodules on the opposite side in mirror image. The patient has no complaints. The most likely diagnosis is

 (A) metastatic squamous cell carcinoma
 (B) reactive lymph node hyperplasia
 (C) fibrous scar
 (D) varicosities at ligated tributaries of the excised jugular
 (E) neuromas

ANSWERS AND TUTORIALS ON ITEMS 399-408

The answers are: **399-C; 400-C; 401-B; 402-C; 403-A; 404-A; 405-B; 406-E; 407-E; 408-E**.

399. This description is that of a thyroglossal duct cyst. These may occasionally become inflamed as it appears to have recently in this instance, and antibiotic therapy will not cause its complete resolution, since the embryologic abnormality remains even when the inflammation subsides. Incision and drainage will not be adequate therapy, and may produce a fistula which will persist so long as the cells remain in the embryologic development track. Simple excision is inadequate, since the extent goes from the base of the tongue through the hyoid bone to the thyroid gland, and incision must be carried out to the base of the tongue and include the midportion of the hyoid if recurrence is to be avoided (Sistrunk procedure).

It is not an uncommon congenital abnormality with no likelihood of malignancy at the time of this girl's presentation, and unlike pharyngeal arch abnormalities, there should be no associated anomalies of the ear. Because of its attachment from the foramen cecum, motion of the tongue such as protrusion or swallowing causes the cyst to move its position in the neck, an observation that can confirm its origin in the thyroglossal duct.

400. The reliability of this finding is somewhat dependent on the observance of the patient, but if that seems trustworthy, it is unlikely to be malignant. The "rule of sevens" is a reference to this, that if a lesion has been present seven days it is inflammatory, seven months it is malignant, seven years it is congenital. Alcoholism and tobacco use are the highest correlations, and radiation at a very young age would be even more suspicious than therapeutic radiation for acne in the teenage years which is less likely to produce thyroid malignancy, but is, nonetheless, a risk factor.

Smoking is probably the most highly correlated risk factor, and that would include a cumulative risk even if recent cessation had followed an earlier history. It is obvious that metastatic spread can occur from a tumor elsewhere, but the presence of a known tumor elsewhere in the body additionally increases the likelihood of a new primary cancer found in the head and neck region.

401. There is no point to cervical splinting in a patient who has lost the strut that tethers the tongue anteriorly, since the tongue will fall back with or without cervical extension in the absence of the mandibular arch. Cricothyroidotomy is a temporizing procedure, and the patient is going to require tracheostomy both immediately and for the foreseeable future because of the multiple injury, anticipated swelling, and loss of bony support as well as soft tissue trauma.

Extension of the neck is also contraindicated until the status of the cervical spine is determined. Nasal catheterization for oxygen delivery will be ineffective if the obstruction is in the pharynx where the swollen tongue has fallen back. Hyperextension of the neck as is required for endotracheal intubation would cause the tongue to fall back during that process, which also puts at risk the cervical spine which is as yet unevaluated. Tracheostomy is both the first and last indicated procedure for securing this patient's airway.

402. This is over-treatment for the T-1 size laryngeal cancer in the larynx, since the presentation of laryngeal cancer is often early because of changes in the voice marking a sensitive indication for screening. Radiotherapy may be the preferred treatment, but laser laryngoscopy with repeated follow-up to detect the occurrence of any new nodules, benign or malignant, may be a second choice. If that has already occurred, then a partial excision or hemilaryngectomy is the appropriate treatment, but total laryngectomy with loss of the larynx for voice purposes is reserved for larger tumor sizes which cannot be treated by these more conservative limited means.

403. In a surprise reversal for head and neck tumors in the adult, the majority of parotid tumors are benign. In fact, in comparison with the other salivary glands, the obverse is true in that 80% of tumors arising in these glands are malignant, a fact probably designed purely for test-taking purposes! The primary parotid tumors can grow to be huge, and although facial nerve palsy suggests malignancy, benign tumors may also give the same feature; neither the nerve palsy nor extension into the deep lobe are contraindications to resection. Surgical therapy is the treatment, although even the benign tumors have a recurrence rate that is high, but radiation therapy is not a successful curative treatment, and is unlikely to be indicated for the vast majority of benign parotid tumors.

404. There is an important distinction to be made between vocal polyps and vocal nodules. Vocal polyps are unilateral. They are not typically associated with voice abuse and do not respond to speech therapy, and require operation, probably in contemporary practice with laser treatment. Vocal nodules are bilateral lesions at the "kissing" contact points at the anterior junction between the front and middle thirds of each vocal chord. The voice lessons can help resolve this by decreasing stress to this area, and surgery is rarely indicated for these "singer's nodules".

405. Malignancy is a very high likelihood given this patient's presentation. However, there are distinctive differences that might lead to consideration of other diagnoses. The presentation is not at all typical for thyroid cancer. The patient is unlikely to have a congenital abnormality that first presents in adult life with this amount of inflammation, even if alcoholism and debilitation may contribute to weakened defenses. Squamous cell carcinoma is a very highly likely possibility, but at least one unsuccessful attempt was made to confirm this. It may have been missed, but it is not typical for epidermoid carcinoma to give draining sinuses. Radiation may contribute to tissue necrosis and ulceration, and devitalized tissue may constitute foreign body nidus with a continuing drainage. There is a strong inflammatory component to this, and in the patient's suppressed state any number of etiologic agents that might not cause disease in someone with good nutrition might become pathogenic.

In this case, the diagnosis turns out to be atypical tuberculosis. In this instance, antimicrobial therapy is not as useful as complete excision of the draining sinus tracks to eliminate the local focus of infection which is serving as a foreign body nidus to the giant cell reaction. Draining cervical lymphadenitis has the term "scrofula" applied to it as well as the delightful historic reference of the "King's Evil" since the touch of the king was supposed to relieve the patient of this problem; it certainly would if that touch is extended to curettage and excision of the involved cervical lymphadenitis!

406. Any of the more radical treatments advised should be applied quickly before the lesion goes away! Particularly in this cosmetically sensitive location, no disfigurement from excision, grafting, radiation (and its associated risks to growth and later carcinogenesis) or permanent cosmetic cover should be attempted. Embolization would not be very easy given the possible feeding vessels, and spontaneous thrombosis is likely without this manipulation. Parents are also to be told that local manipulation (compressing it with taped-on coins, heat, cold, or daily cosmetic application) would perhaps do more to induce the self-consciousness that they are concerned about than the ongoing devolution of what is a transient stage in this lesion. There is a role for tattooing of permanent cosmetic features such as some "port-wine stains". But for the cavernous hemangioma the appropriate treatment is the passage of time.

407. Tonsillectomy is not indicated for tonsillitis in children, but it may be for the complications of tonsillitis. Tonsillitis is a primary indication for antibiotic treatment and local management for symptomatic relief. However, there are complications that stem from secondary infectious sequelae, such as peritonsillar abscess or an allergy from resident bacteria or upper air or food passage disruption based on a mass effect from very hypertrophic tonsils.

In times past, six patients with the same last name would be posted sequentially on the OR schedule with a homey note in the hospital news bulletin with a caption under a photograph saying something like "the family Robinson is having its tonsils removed today". This gimmickry is inappropriate, since tonsils do not need removing because they are there. Even primary pathology is not an indication, unless there is a second order phenomenon that would justify this procedure with a benefit that is anticipated to outweigh the risk.

408. Along the posterior border of the field of radical neck dissection, the cervical plexus of cutaneous nerves is encountered in the segmental distribution from auricular nerves inferiorly. These are each sectioned in turn as expendable, with attention directed to the preservation of cranial nerves to the extent possible, a necessity for certain nerves such as the vagus and desirable for the spinal accessory nerve which is not sectioned unless necessary and with the consequent disability of the "winged scapula". This sectioning produces neuromas that are rarely hypersensitive and usually are sensitive only for a short time. They may be confused with lymph nodes (which should mostly have been cleared in the dissection bloc) or metastatic deposits but their anatomic regularity makes them more easily recognized as benign consequences of the radical neck dissection. Ligated vein tributaries shrivel following thrombosis, and postoperative scarring would not be so anatomically regular in this pattern.

Items 409-418

409. Each of the following conditions is a primary indication for thyroidectomy **EXCEPT**:

   (A) thyroiditis
   (B) two cm thyroid nodule with hoarseness
   (C) recurrent Graves' disease in second trimester pregnancy
   (D) dysphagia with submanubrial goiter
   (E) positive fine needle aspirate cytology

410. Which of the following studies is both necessary and sufficient in the absence of other compelling clinical features to indicate thyroidectomy?

   (A) technetium scan
   (B) iodine scan
   (C) ultrasound
   (D) arteriogram
   (E) fine needle aspiration cytology

411. Each of the following statements is true regarding a two cm differentiated papillary thyroid cancer in a 24 year-old woman **EXCEPT**:

   (A) involvement of adjacent cervical lymph nodes with papillary cancer changes the staging of the primary tumor with a worse prognosis
   (B) tumor free survival rate following treatment is expected at greater than 90% in ten years
   (C) radical neck dissection should not be combined with total thyroidectomy from the side of the lobe with the primary tumor
   (D) such a nodule is most often cold on scan
   (E) operation is elective and could be postponed four weeks on the basis of patient's request that it not interfere with a personal matter she does not care to divulge

412. Which of the following lesions in the thyroid is typically unifocal with unlikely disease elsewhere in the thyroid gland?

   (A) Plummer's syndrome
   (B) medullary thyroid cancer in a teenager
   (C) follicular carcinoma
   (D) papillary carcinoma
   (E) *struma lymphomatosa*

413. Each of the following statements concerning medullary thyroid cancer is true **EXCEPT**:

   (A) it may occur in families with a genetic predisposition for it
   (B) it is nearly always multicentric when found in young patients
   (C) radioiodine treatment is the therapy of choice for control of lymph node metastases
   (D) metastatic disease in the liver, lungs or regional spread can be detected in the absence of imaging studies by characteristic secretions from the tumor
   (E) the prognosis following surgical treatment is much worse than that for papillary carcinoma of comparable stage

414. Which of the following statements regarding follicular thyroid carcinoma is true?

   (A) its incidence is highest in populations where iodine deficiency is widespread
   (B) prevalence of follicular carcinoma in the United States has increased remarkably in this century
   (C) it is the most common cancer found in patients who report a history of head and neck irradiation
   (D) multicentricity is the rule rather than the exception
   (E) lymphatic metastases are a principle means of spread

415. Which of the following tumor cell types has the worst prognosis in the thyroid gland?

    (A) lymphoma
    (B) anaplastic carcinoma
    (C) medullary carcinoma
    (D) papillary carcinoma
    (E) follicular carcinoma

416. A young man with follicular carcinoma of the thyroid treated by total thyroidectomy is asymptomatic, but follow-up scan when he has been off thyroid replacement shows bilateral pulmonary uptake of the isotope. Which of the following statements is true regarding this condition?

    (A) this distribution is an artifact, and there is no confirmed evidence of metastasis until lung biopsy is carried out
    (B) the patient is doomed to a very short life expectancy from this heavy metastatic tumor burden
    (C) wedge resections of lung should be undertaken in bilateral staged thoracotomies to reduce the bulk of the pulmonary metastases
    (D) following radioiodine therapy, prolonged tumor-free survival is anticipated
    (E) chemotherapy should be initiated with cytotoxic drugs used in combination

417. Which of the following characteristics of a patient with thyroid cancer has the most effect on prognosis?

    (A) degree of differentiation
    (B) tumor stage
    (C) lymph node involvement
    (D) tumor size
    (E) patient's age

418. Each of the following complications of subtotal thyroidectomy for Graves' disease is unique to operative treatment and does not occur with radioiodine **EXCEPT**:

    (A) hemorrhage
    (B) hypoparathyroidism
    (C) hypothyroidism
    (D) recurrent laryngeal nerve injury
    (E) superior laryngeal nerve injury

ANSWERS AND TUTORIALS ON ITEMS 409-418

The answers are: **409-A; 410-E; 411-A; 412-C; 413-C; 414-A; 415-B; 416-D; 417-E; 418-C**.

409. Thyroiditis may cause hyperthyroidism when, early in its course, it stimulates production and release of thyroid hormones (so-called Hashimoto's toxic thyroiditis), but inflammatory processes in the thyroid are usually self-limited, and often result in a "burnout" in the end-stage. The patient may experience some discomfort, but this can be handled with <u>analgesics and anti-inflammatories</u>, and thyroid operation would likely only speed up the onset of hypothyroidism. This problem is more common in (women) and is getting increasingly more frequent for reasons that are not known. Treatment is most generally symptomatic if there is some degree of hyperfunction, and long-term thyroid replacement is the treatment in the hypothyroid later stages of fibrosis. The presence of, or high probability of, thyroid malignancy is an indication for operation, and <u>fine needle aspiration cytology</u> has refined that possibility to a probability. Clinical evidence is still useful, however, and hoarseness with a thyroid nodule that has caused either recurrent laryngeal paralysis or laryngeal invasion is indicative of malignancy with or without cytologic confirmation.

Compression of the upper air or food passages is strong indication for relief of the compression, as is most frequently the case with goiters with large expanding intrathoracic components inside enclosure that compromises the airway. The patient with recurrent Graves' disease is an appropriate candidate for surgery, particularly if pregnant. These conditions are "staples" in thyroid surgery, but must be distinguished from the larger number of benign goiters that will not require surgical treatment.

410. Each of the radiographic imaging studies constitute "shadow producing procedures". That the thyroid nodule occupies space is likely known already from the clinical examination since that is the presentation of most thyroid nodules. Further information about this mass is limited in knowing its blood flow (technetium and arteriography) or its iodine concentration ability (iodine scan). The ultrasound can tell us whether it is solid or cystic, information strongly suggested on clinical examination as well, and none of the diagnostic studies just mentioned would give opportunity for treatment simultaneously as would needle aspiration in the event that the lesion turned out to be cystic. Since the information yield has not been critical (i.e., malignant lesions can be hot or cold, relatively more or less vascular, and some have cystic degeneration) the only value added to the information obtained in imaging is a microscopic appreciation of the nature of the mass.

Cutting tissue with a core needle biopsy could give histology which is helpful, but a more rapid assessment can be done with cytology through fine needle aspiration, which is now the method of choice for the assessment of a thyroid nodule based on clinical features that recommend its cytologic identification, generally now in preference to one of the shadow producing procedures, since much more value is added than a confirmation that the mass can be imaged.

411. It comes as a surprise to many who are accustomed to the staging systems for adenocarcinomas elsewhere that cervical lymph node involvement does not change papillary thyroid cancer staging. The prognosis is not impaired by lymph node involvement, and lymph node status does not significantly alter treatment. That the nodes were found to be involved is likely because they were taken with the thyroidectomy specimen, and residual cellular disease not excised is likely to be ablated by radioiodine follow-up in the absence of the "iodine sink" when the thyroid is gone. This treatment does not need to be combined with radical neck dissection, and this therapy would result in excess of 90% disease free survival long-term. These nodules are not invariably cold, although they tend to be, since differentiated thyroid cancer frequently concentrates iodine, and in fact, that is the basis of radioiodine follow-up therapy. This usually requires enhanced TSH, which also occurs naturally after thyroidectomy if thyroid replacement is withheld until radio-iodine adjunctive administration. Operation can be scheduled electively, and there is every reason to honor the patient's request, since there is negligible risk of tumor spread in the interval suggested.

412. Plummer's syndrome is the hyperfunctioning of an autonomous nodule in a preexisting multinodular goiter. Since nearly all of the thyroid gland is involved with the multinodular goiter, this disqualifies this benign condition as it does *struma lymphomatosa* which is chronic thyroiditis of the Hashimoto type, affecting all parts of the thyroid in inflammation. Familial medullary thyroid carcinoma originates in both lobes wherever parafollicular C-cells are scattered in their multicentric malignant degeneration. Papillary carcinoma is more often than not multicentric, which is one of the rationales employed in advocating at least lobectomy and probably thyroidectomy to eradicate the other foci of the disease besides the primary presenting nodule. Of the lesions listed, only follicular carcinoma typically stands alone, and it may arise in an otherwise normal thyroid gland.

413. Medullary thyroid cancer originates from C-cells, which are parafollicular and do not iodinate thyronine. Therefore, whether inside or out of the thyroid in lymphatic or other locations, concentration of radioiodine does not occur and radioiodine therapy for lymphatic metastases would be ineffective. It can occur in families, and when it does so, younger affected patients have nearly always multicentric disease. It can be found by stimulated release of calcitonin in response to calcium or pentagastrin through venous catheters positioned for sampling from potential metastatic sites. Its prognosis is much poorer than papillary carcinoma in even the most advanced stage of the latter in comparison with even earlier stages of the former, since spread is early and aggressive in most instances, and especially so in the hereditary type called MEA-IIB.

414. Because follicular carcinoma is associated with iodine deficiency, the widespread use of iodized salt in the United States has caused a remarkable decrease in the incidence of follicular cancer within this century. Unlike papillary carcinoma, in which multicentricity is the rule, follicular carcinomas are usually unifocal. They spread by capsular and vascular invasion, and lymphatic metastases are not a prominent method of metastases. The most common form of cancer discovered in patients who have reported head and neck irradiation is papillary carcinoma although follicular carcinomas may rarely be seen in such patients.

415. Anaplastic carcinoma is essentially an untreatable disease, with nearly uniformly fatal outcome despite the treatments that have been tried. It spreads quickly and early and is not controlled by radioiodine, radiation or chemotherapy. Extensive surgical efforts have resulted in some relief of obstructive disease while tumor spread usually continues unchecked. In order of malignant behavior, medullary thyroid carcinoma would be next worst, followed by follicular, lymphoma (which may present primarily in the thyroid gland) and papillary with the best prognosis.

416. In very fortunate contrast to other tumors such as sarcoma that might spread by the hematogenous route to fill the lungs with metastases, this form of thyroid cancer has a good prognosis, due largely to the "magic bullet" of iodine concentration in the thyroid tissue that can be further enhanced with the TSH stimulation that occurs naturally in hypothyroidism. This directed "smart weapon" is magnified in the "homing signal" provided by that iodine concentrating capacity that is evident in the uptake of this metastatic disease. It is unlikely to be present in small pulmonary nodules in the pattern of sarcoma spread, so bilateral thoracotomy for the purpose of metastatic wedge resection would be futile, and unnecessary given the superior treatment results with radioiodine. Cytotoxic chemotherapy has not proven effective in thyroid cancer and would not be given.

417. The biologic factors predominate in prognosis of thyroid cancers and many of them are "given" rather than controllable. The single most important is the patient's age, since if all other features were held constant, the younger patient has a better prognosis. Lymph node involvement, as previously noted, is not a principle factor in changing the staging of tumors of the same size, but size is a factor, and staging is principally determined by T-stage with much less contribution from N-staging. Differentiation of the tumor for a given cell type, such as papillary, is a significant prognostic factor for groups of patients, but is not as significant as age. Since most of the patients have well differentiated tumors, it is also humbling to note that one prognostic factor absent as a principle determinant of how well patients do is treatment, about which each clinician carries such passionate belief that it is difficult to test treatment options to determine a superior method which we honestly do not know.

418. Hypothyroidism is a condition that may follow Graves' disease whether treated or not and by any means. The hypothyroidism that follows operation is usually within the period of postoperative follow-up, and is recognized and treated by replacement hormone. The hypothyroidism that follows radioiodine, if effective, is nearly inevitable but usually occurs much later than the follow-up period, and is often insidious and untreated. In fact, late hypothyroidism is the chief disadvantage of radioiodine therapy that does accomplish the control of hyperthyroidism without recurrence. One of the principle advantages to operation is its low incidence of hypothyroidism after surgical therapy, and operation should be preferred since drug-free follow-up and autoregulation of the pituitary-thyroid axis is possible. The surgical complications of hemorrhage, hypoparathyroidism from disturbance of the parathyroid glands or their blood supply, and dysfunction of either superior or recurrent laryngeal nerves is more likely to happen with surgery than radioiodine. However, it should be noted that recurrent laryngeal nerve palsy has happened following radioiodine treatment, and has been reported, even bilaterally, simply with intubation in a patient undergoing operation outside the neck or chest.

Items 419-428

419. Which of the following statements is true concerning the parathyroid glands and is useful in identifying them in their embryologically possible ectopic positions?

    (A) blood supply of the superior parathyroid usually originates from the superior thyroid artery, and the blood supply of the inferior parathyroid usually arises from the inferior thyroid artery
    (B) the inferior parathyroid gland originates in association with a pharyngeal pouch superior to the superior parathyroid gland's origin
    (C) neither superior nor inferior parathyroid glands descend into the neck if the thyroid doesn't
    (D) the parathyroid is derived from neuroectoderm
    (E) the parathyroid glands have no embryologic relationship to the thymus

420. Which of the following lesions is **LEAST** common?

    (A) parathyroid cyst
    (B) parathyroid hyperplasia
    (C) chief cell adenoma
    (D) parathyroid carcinoma
    (E) oxyphil cell adenoma

421. The most typical presentation of the hypercalcemic patients proven by operation to have primary hyperparathyroidism currently is

    (A) asymptomatic
    (B) renal stones
    (C) bone pain and radiographic evidence of resorption
    (D) abdominal pain
    (E) disorientation and change in personality

422. One unusual familial syndrome that may be confused with primary hyperparathyroidism which it closely mimics can be distinguished by urinary calcium determination in hypercalcemic patients. This syndrome is

    (A) secondary hyperparathyroidism
    (B) tertiary hyperparathyroidism
    (C) sarcoidosis
    (D) hypocalciuric hypercalcemia
    (E) renal tubular acidosis

423. After the confident biochemical and endocrine confirmation of primary hyperparathyroidism in the hypercalcemic patient, which of the following studies is required before parathyroid exploration is first attempted?

    (A) thallium-technetium scanning
    (B) none
    (C) ultrasonography
    (D) thyrocervical angiography
    (E) selective venous sampling for parathormone

424. Total thyroidectomy is an operation frequently carried out, but total parathyroidectomy should be avoided at some considerable effort. The principle reason for this is

    (A) total parathyroidectomy has a much higher risk to the recurrent laryngeal nerves
    (B) there is no satisfactory replacement for endogenous parathormone
    (C) ablation of the parathyroid glands endangers the blood supply to the anterior cervical spinal cord
    (D) parathyroidectomy is too technically difficult, and can only be done with an operating microscope
    (E) cancer develops in the thyroid gland more frequently than in the parathyroid glands

425. Each of the following surgical procedures is appropriate for secondary hyperparathyroidism **EXCEPT**:

    (A) excision of three and a half parathyroid glands
    (B) excision of one large parathyroid gland and biopsy of a second
    (C) reduction of all discoverable parathyroid tissue down to approximately 100 mg in residual well vascularized tissue
    (D) total parathyroidectomy from all cervical and mediastinal locations and autograft of small portions of one gland in forearm muscle
    (E) renal transplantation and observation to see if secondary hyperparathyroidism resolves

426. In all patients in the US who might be demonstrated to have hypercalcemia, the single most prevalent cause is

   (A) primary hyperparathyroidism
   (B) secondary hyperparathyroidism
   (C) malignancy
   (D) milk-alkali syndrome
   (E) hyperthyroidism

427. The most frequent cause of failure of a primary cervical exploration to correct primary hyperparathyroidism is

   (A) regrowth of subtotally resected parathyroid tissue in secondary hyperparathyroidism
   (B) parathyroidosis
   (C) parathyroid carcinoma
   (D) failure to appreciate multiple gland disease
   (E) familial hypocalciuric hypercalcemia

428. Postoperative hypocalcemia immediately following parathyroid exploration strongly suggests which of the following is true?

   (A) the surgeon has probably excised or devascularized all the parathyroid tissue
   (B) if the patient is asymptomatic, low calcium numbers are not treated, but uncomfortable complaints are managed with calcium replacement
   (C) this condition is an indication for parathyroid allograft
   (D) the patient should receive vitamin D treatment as soon as the serum calcium fall below 10 mg/dl
   (E) unlike hypercalcemia, bone or joint discomfort is *not* a clinical feature in this form of hypocalcemia

ANSWERS AND TUTORIALS ON ITEMS 419-428

The answers are: **419-B; 420-D; 421-A; 422-D; 423-B; 424-B; 425-B; 426-C; 427-D; 428-B**.

419. The parathyroid glands peregrinate around the neck and mediastinum in embryologic development, but they have to carry their blood supply with them, and usually they have a predictable pattern of unpredictability in location. The search for the anatomically possible position, is helped by knowing which gland it is that appears missing. The inferior parathyroid gland has actually descended further from its embryologic origin, and sometimes does not stop in the customary position, but continues on down into the thymic tongue into the mediastinum. When it does so, its blood supply can frequently be identified as a tether dragged behind it, branching from the inferior thyroid artery. The inferior thyroid artery supplies both superior and inferior parathyroid glands, and typically the side on which an enlarged parathyroid gland is located is quickly approximated by the relative size of the inferior thyroid arteries. An enlarged gland also has an enlarged feeding vessel, and it is helpful to follow such an apparent vessel bound into the mediastinum in the event that the inferior parathyroid gland is missing. It is also surgically significant that the chest does not need to be opened, since the arterial control will remain in the neck at the level of the inferior thyroid artery while teasing back the wayward parathyroid gland from its mediastinal hiding place.

420. In the United States, parathyroid carcinoma is remarkably rare, at least as it may present as hyperparathyroidism. It is rarer still when the criterion of diagnosis is metastatic disease that can cause the patient's death. For some reason, there is a much higher incidence in Japan, although some would doubt the clinical significance of this because of the use of different histopathologic criteria. Parathyroid cyst is somewhat more common if the degenerated adenomas with cystic features following involution, often accompanied by hypercalcemic crises, are added. Oxyphil adenoma is rare, and the majority of hyperparathyroidism is based in chief cell hyperplasia. Both hyperplastic oxyphil cell and chief cell tissue cannot be distinguished in a single specimen from a process called adenoma in one gland. In the confusion between the terms two gland hyperplasia or double adenomas becomes futile. The best description for hyperfunctioning parathyroid tissue is that it exists in single or multiple gland disease.

421. Hyperparathyroidism is now nearly uniformly found as an incidental biochemical abnormality on screening blood examination. It is probably the most valuable yield of the multichannel autoanalyzer, since hypercalcemia is always worth investigation for discovery of diseases that are either treatable, significant with respect to prognosis, or when correction would prevent further problems. The old mnemonic "stones, bones, moans, and abdominal groans" defines the past pattern of advance stage disease which brought patients to have these complaints investigated. Retrospectively, there is some insidious loss of capability (forgetfulness, headache, many features attributed to advancing age) that are only recognized by their absence when hyperparathyroidism is relieved. However, the minority of patients now present with one of the major complications, and asymptomatic population screening with a rapid, relatively inexpensive and reliable method has found the indicators that are proven to be related to the illness. These findings in asymptomatic patients raise the question of whether the disease is being treated in advance of its appearance other than by biochemical markers when it might not ever cause symptomatic disease. This is often resolved in favor of operation for those with an arbitrarily selected higher value of serum calcium concentration than for those with lower levels of elevation, unless any early clinical features appear to be developing.

422. A familial syndrome has been discovered in patients who have had failed parathyroid explorations for persistent hypercalcemia, until it is found that they have lower urinary excretion of calcium based in a higher "setpoint" for renal threshold for circulating calcium.

Hyperparathyroidism is appropriate stimulation of the parathyroid glands, usually from chronic renal failure and hyperphosphatemia. If such patients are transplanted and renal failure resolves, persistent hyperparathyroidism is referred to as tertiary when the reactive hyperparathyroidism of secondary form turns autonomous. Sarcoidosis is, in effect, a hypersensitivity to vitamin D, and renal tubular acidosis is part of the differential diagnosis of hypercalcemia, but has none of the other features of hyperparathyroidism.

423. Of the most sensitive tests for identifying the surgical objective — that is normal or suppressed parathyroid glands which may be much smaller than any radiographic imaging threshold — the primary surgical exploration is the only method that is satisfactory in all and successful in most. The reliability of each radiographic method listed is less than that of most experienced surgeons, and considerably less than experienced endocrine surgeons who are frequently called upon to perform re-exploratory surgery. In these instances, imaging and selective sampling can be most helpful in limiting exploration, not only to find the hyperfunctioning parathyroid tissue, but what is more important to the long-term benefit of the patient, to avoid destruction of residual parathyroid tissue that might be restored to normal function. None of the imaging tests are needed before primary cervical exploration, and a selective approach to only those tests needed to guide re-exploration is appropriate for re-operative work.

424. A patient who is aparathyroid is suffering a crippling disorder with continuous requirement of vitamin D and calcium to inadequately maintain a serum calcium always dangerously close to tetany levels. The other technical and biologic reasons listed are trivial for the technical reasons and false in the biologic assertions. It is true that thyroid cancer is more prevalent than parathyroid cancer, but that would not mean total ablation of all parathyroid glands, since it is usually a unifocal disease, and ablation of the other parathyroids does not enhance the uptake of any given treatment directed at the parathyroid. Total parathyroidectomy or its functional equivalent by interrupting its blood supply is altogether too easy, and is sometimes unintentionally performed in total thyroidectomy (which might more appropriately be called a "parathyroid preservation procedure").

425. Secondary hyperparathyroidism is a disease in which all glands should be appropriately responding to the hyperphosphatemia by hyperplasia. It is, simply, multiglandular disease, so the search for a single hyperfunctioning gland and confirmation of the presence of another is — as it would be in most instances of primary hyperparathyroidism that are sporadic (except — notably — any familial disease) — inappropriate treatment in secondary hyperparathyroidism. Two of the responses show reduction of the excessive parathyroid tissue down to a level that should give function without hyperfunction — one of those leaving half of one gland, and the other attempting to leave at least two sites on intact vasculature but not to exceed 100 mg in total. In very experienced hands, total parathyroidectomy with careful preservation and transplantation techniques have been able to eradicate parathyroid tissue from the neck, and place it in a position where it can not only "take", but in many instances, again become hyperplastic and result in hyperfunction, but in this instance can be reduced by re-excision of the implanted fragments under local anesthesia as an outpatient. It is also possible to treat secondary hyperparathyroidism expectantly, if the primary stimulus to its hyperplastic stimulus response is corrected as with transplantation. If the hyperfunction continues after phosphate clearances improve, this situation is referred to as tertiary hyperparathyroidism, and in this instance of autonomy is treated, once again, as primary hyperparathyroidism.

426. Hypercalcemia is a common and vexing complication of some of the most common types of visceral malignancy, and shortens life and increases morbidity in patients who suffer from it. This especially includes breast cancer, but may also include lung cancer, hypernephroma, prostate cancer, each representing tumors with a predilection for bone metastases. It is for this reason that it was stated earlier that hypercalcemia is always a significant pickup on multichannel blood tests, in this instance because of its prognostic significance and management requirement rather that potential for cure. Most patients with secondary hyperparathyroidism would not be suffering from an unknown condition since most of them are on dialysis. Sarcoidosis and milk-alkali syndrome can give hypercalcemia, and hyperthyroidism can also. One group of patients in whom the hypercalcemia may be the first indication of any illness since they are otherwise asymptomatic would be the patients with primary hyperparathyroidism, and this group runs a close second behind malignancy in prevalence in hypercalcemic patients.

427. Multiple gland disease that is treated as though it were primary hyperparathyroidism based in single gland pathology is the source of failure in most primary cervical explorations that do not control hypercalcemia. The patient who is at risk for this undertreatment is the patient with secondary hyperparathyroidism in which there may be supernumerary glands, that is, more than the four identified and three and a half that were excised. This is nearly always the case in familial hyperparathyroidism, since multiple gland disease is the rule. If the first enlarged parathyroid encountered is removed, and another less imposing gland identified as "normal", this patient will have recurrence, if not persistence. Persistence is referred to as hypercalcemia that is present within six months of the operation (usually it is obvious on the same day) and recurrence refers to hypercalcemia that follows operation by more than six months during which hypercalcemia is absent. Parathyroid carcinoma may spread and hyperfunction, but it is rare to begin with, and rarer still that it would be a source of persistent hypercalcemia. FHH might be a source of failure when operation is done on a propositus of a kindred as yet unknown, but testing urinary calcium clearance in this patient should identify hypercalcemic relatives who have the same problem. As yet, this syndrome — although reported in many families — is cumulatively not large enough to account for a clinically significant number of primary parathyroid operation failures.

428. The very hypocalcemia that is expected to result from excision of a large hyperfunctioning parathyroid gland is the signal that would stimulate the hypoplastic parathyroids to recover function normally, so early treatment of hypocalcemia in the absence of patient symptoms is not indicated because it may protract recovery of residual parathyroid secretion. There is a syndrome of postparathyroidectomy arthritis due to pseudogout, so that paradoxically the bone pain that was said to be symptomatic of hypercalcemia may be a complication of its correction early in the hypocalcemic course. It is not likely that all the parathyroid tissue has been destroyed, although that is a remote possibility, and will only be determined when the parathormone secretion doesn't return after a period of hypocalcemic stimulus. Vitamin D therapy would be unnecessary, and would be called for only if a patient required calcium supplementation and that was inadequate alone to relieve hypocalcemic symptoms.

CHAPTER VI
UROGENITAL SURGERY
BREAST SURGERY

Items 429-431

An 82 year-old woman is brought from a nursing home with abrupt onset of nausea and vomiting. The irreducible groin mass shown in **Figure 6.1** is discovered on physical examination. It had not been noted at the time of nursing home admission eight months earlier.

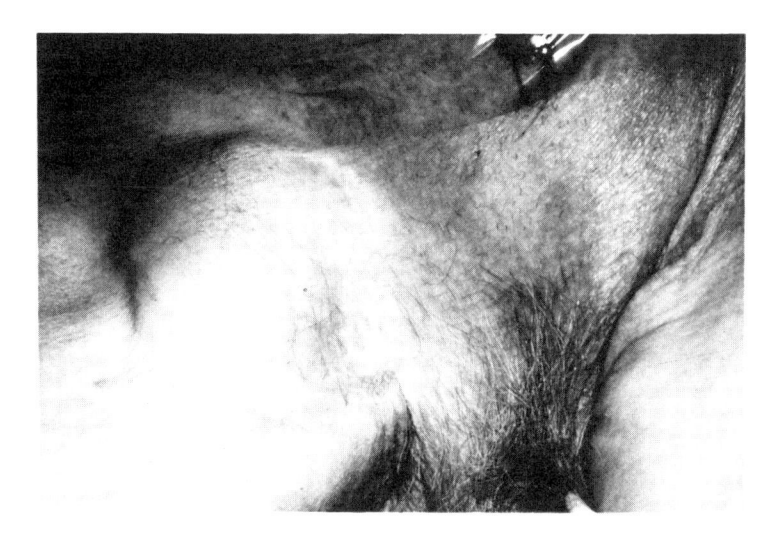

Figure 6.1

429. True statements about this kind of groin mass include

    (A)   it is more common in women than in men
    (B)   it is most often incarcerated
    (C)   it does not require surgical repair
    (D)   it most often has a sliding component
    (E)   it is usually malignant

430. Treatment of this condition should be

    (A) a truss
    (B) an urgent operation
    (C) laparoscopy
    (D) colonoscopy
    (E) vascular resection and prosthesis

431. The complication most likely to happen next if untreated would be

    (A) hemorrhage
    (B) perforation
    (C) complete bowel obstruction
    (D) malignant degeneration
    (E) thrombosis

ANSWERS AND TUTORIAL ON ITEMS 429-431

The answers are: **429-A; 430-B; 431-C**.

This patient has a femoral hernia, and it is true that they are more common in women than in men, even though indirect inguinal hernia is more common than femoral hernia in women because of higher frequency overall. Femoral hernias may incarcerate, and do so more frequently than indirect inguinal hernias. Not all femoral hernias present as incarceration. However, incarceration does require urgent surgical repair and not management with some other means such as a truss. Bowel obstruction, progressing to complete obstruction is likely if the full bowel circumference is involved in the hernia rather than the partial thickness found in a Richter's hernia.

Items 432-434

A 19 year-old woman is seen in the emergency room with right lower quadrant pain, a drop in hematocrit and a positive Gravindex test with last menstrual period 50 days earlier. In sonography of the abdomen, a mass is seen interpreted as an ovarian cyst. At operation the specimen depicted in **Figure 6.2** is removed.

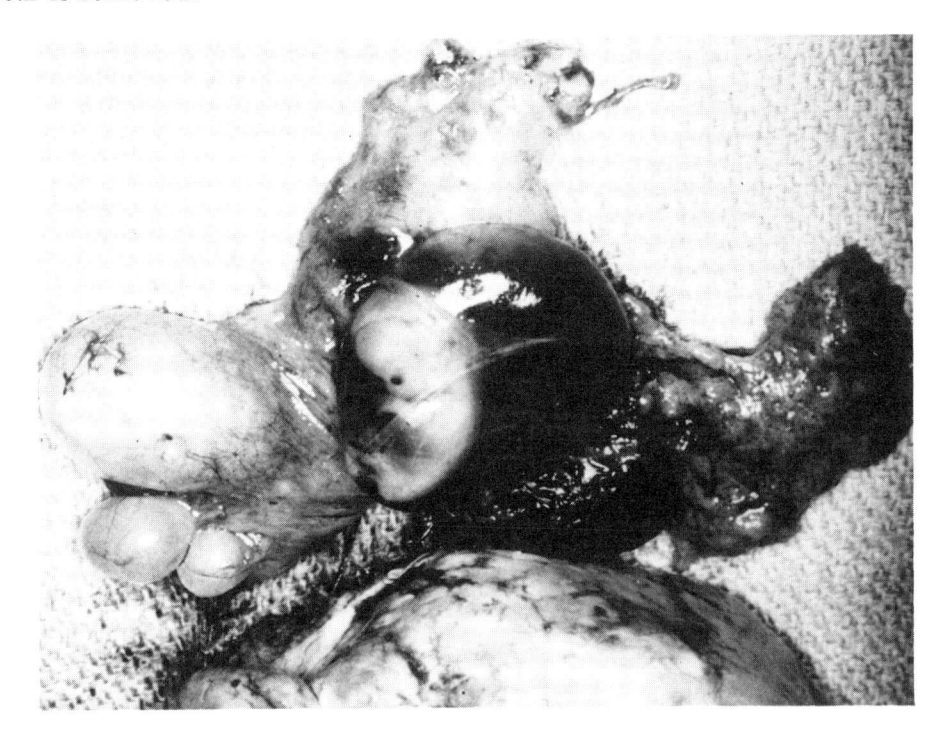

Figure 6.2

432. The nature of the ovarian mass is

    (A) corpus luteum cyst
    (B) teratoma
    (C) adenocarcinoma
    (D) Stein-Leventhal ovary
    (E) endometrioma

433. The risk of highest immediate significance to the patient is

    (A) torsion of the cyst
    (B) hemorrhage
    (C) metastatic spread
    (D) endometriosis
    (E) infertility

434. In the future, the most probable life-threatening risk the patient faces would be

    (A)   tubal abscess
    (B)   torsion ovarian cyst
    (C)   carcinoma of ovary
    (D)   uterine carcinoma
    (E)   ectopic pregnancy

ANSWERS AND TUTORIAL ON ITEMS 432-434

The answers are: **432-A; 433-B; 434-E**.

This patient presents with a finding that should never be ignored in the emergency room and must always be thought of in any reproductive-age female. She has a ruptured ectopic pregnancy. The nature of the ovarian mass is that of corpus luteum cyst, which comes along with the pregnancy. The very vascular nature of a tubal (the most common kind of ectopic) pregnancy with a placental implantation in surrounding tissues makes hemorrhage a very high likelihood and in a volume of bleeding sufficient to cause shock in the patient. With the excision of this tube and adjacent structures, "cross-over" from the opposite ovary to the remaining tube may lead to a higher incidence of ectopic pregnancy in the future following operation for this primary instance of it.

Items 435-437

A 30 year-old woman had a sensation of fullness of the abdomen "like my last pregnancy". A palpable abdominal mass was present. At operation she had the large mass (**Figure 6.3A**) removed and (**Figure 6.3B**) sectioned.

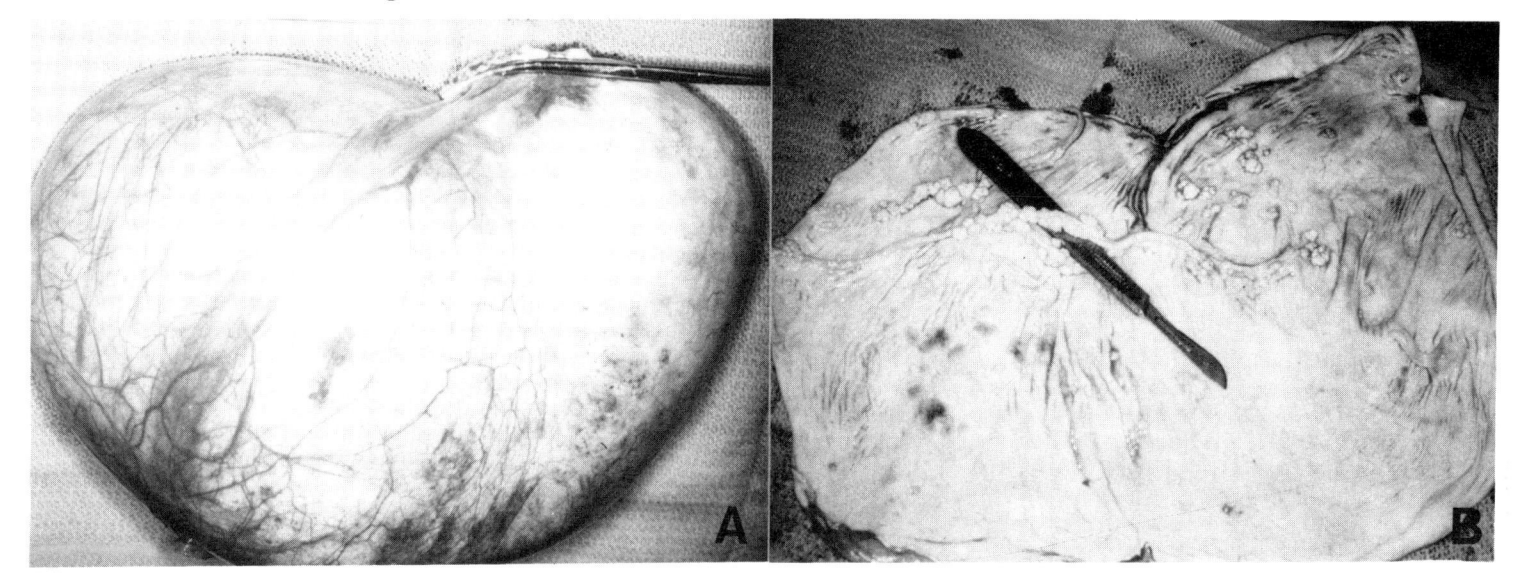

Figure 6.3

435. The mass most likely represents

   (A) cystadenocarcinoma
   (B) simple ovarian cyst
   (C) corpus luteum cyst
   (D) cystic teratoma
   (E) hydatid cyst

436. The most important indication for removal of this mass is to

   (A) prevent malignant degeneration
   (B) decrease likelihood of metastases
   (C) relieve symptoms of mass effect
   (D) prevent rupture and spill of fluid into peritoneum
   (E) prevent torsion

437. In follow-up, the patient should be checked for

- (A) elevated human chorionic gonadotrophin
- (B) malignant ascites
- (C) ectopic pregnancy
- (D) contralateral ovarian cyst development
- (E) daughter cysts throughout peritoneum

ANSWERS AND TUTORIAL ON ITEMS 435-437

The answers are: **435-B; 436-C; 437-D**.

This patient has a very large but simple ovarian cyst. Its very presence gives rise to considerable mass symptoms, and that would be indication for its removal. Following excision of this cyst, contralateral ovarian cyst development must be watched for. However, this is neither infectious nor malignant, and the measures designed for monitoring of patients with either of these conditions are not appropriate for this patient.

Items 438-440

A 20 year-old woman is seen in the emergency room with acute abdominal pain. She is 8 days from her last menstrual period, and has a negative Gravindex. She has a right tender adnexal mass and X-ray shows the outline of a mass with opaque objects on the film within the mass. At operation the mass depicted in **Figure 6.4** is removed.

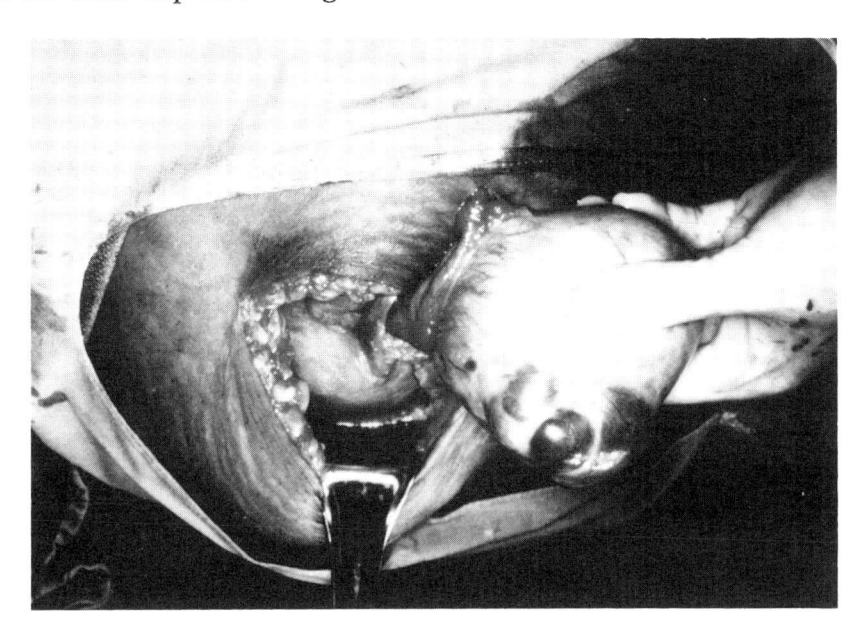

Figure 6.4

438. The most likely diagnosis is

　　(A)　lithopedion
　　(B)　ruptured ectopic pregnancy
　　(C)　torsion ovarian teratoma
　　(D)　infarcted endometrioma
　　(E)　uterine fibroid

439. The opaque objects on X-ray film may likely represent

　　(A)　teeth
　　(B)　fetal bones
　　(C)　calcified fibroid
　　(D)　intrauterine contraceptive device
　　(E)　organizing hematoma

440. The nature of the mass is

   (A) malignant tumor
   (B) infectious cyst
   (C) inflammatory collection
   (D) luteal phase
   (E) benign neoplasm

ANSWERS AND TUTORIAL ON ITEMS 438-440

The answers are: **438-C; 439-A; 440-E**.

This young woman has the classic presentation of ovarian teratoma. The ovarian teratoma is twisted because of its weight and range of positions in the abdomen, giving rise to a torsion of the ovarian teratoma which would be indication for operation. As unlikely as it might seem originally, the opaque objects on the X-ray film would most likely represent teeth! That is because teeth, hair, and other epidermoid structures are fairly common in teratomas, and the teeth are the most radiopaque components and when present can be diagnostic of ovarian teratoma. Although these may have components within each of three germ layers and one or more of these may be malignant, the most common presentation in this age group and under these circumstances is that of a benign neoplasm.

Items 441-443

A 40 year-old woman had a pelvic mass first described as uterine fibroids. With abdominal distension and ascites, this was re-evaluated and operation undertaken with the total abdominal hysterectomy and bilateral salpingo-oophorectomy specimen shown in **Figure 6.5**.

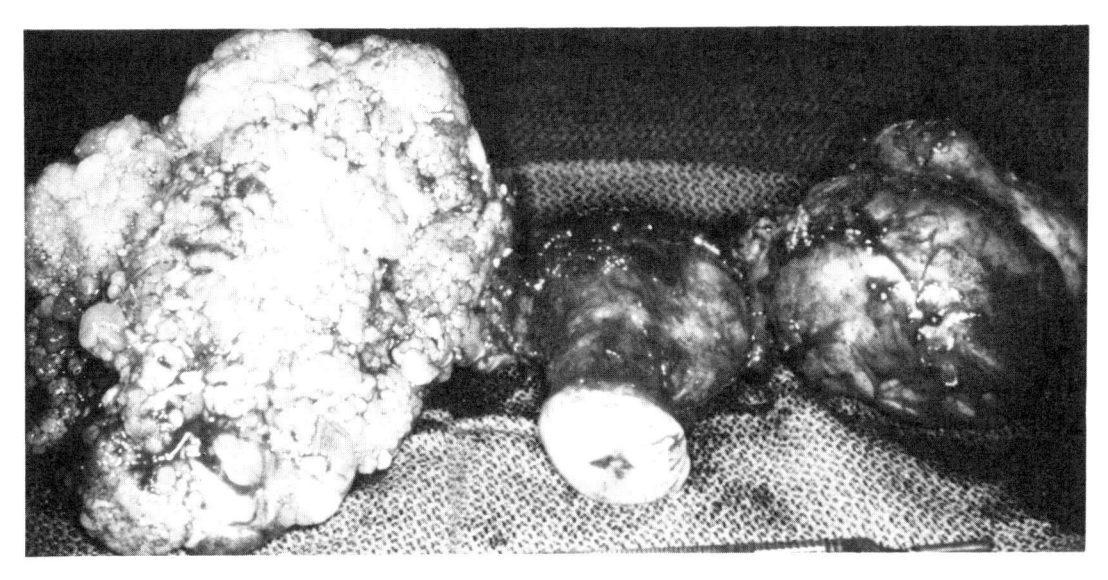

Figure 6.5

441. The specimen shown most likely represents

    (A) bilateral ovarian cysts
    (B) Stage III ovarian carcinoma
    (C) endometriosis
    (D) tubo-ovarian abscess
    (E) ectopic pregnancy

442. Additional components of the operation would include

    (A) omentectomy
    (B) splenectomy
    (C) liver biopsy
    (D) colostomy
    (E) hepatic artery cannulation

443. The follow-up pattern predicted for the patient is

    (A)   very low likelihood of response to chemotherapy
    (B)   high response to chemotherapy and 90% 5 year survival
    (C)   30% response to chemotherapy and 60% 5 year survival
    (D)   high initial response to chemotherapy but early recurrence
    (E)   60% response to radiotherapy and 60% 5 year survival

ANSWERS AND TUTORIAL ON ITEMS 441-443

The answers are: **441-B; 442-A; 443-D**.

This patient has bilateral ovarian adenocarcinoma presenting in Stage III. In addition to the total abdominal hysterectomy and removal of both ovaries and tubes, omentectomy is an additional component of the operation, since ovarian carcinoma is really a disease of the peritoneum. Debulking as much tumor as can be found in addition to that which is located within the gynecologic organs would be helpful in order to get the best effect of chemotherapy. Chemotherapy is likely to produce a favorable response rate initially, and despite this very high initial response rate to chemotherapy, early recurrence is likely, with a limited prognosis following the chemotherapy which will be used as an adjunct to this operation.

Items 444-446

A gravida 3, para 2 woman enters labor with normal delivery of a 8 pound Apgar 9 infant. The afterbirth is spontaneously passed, although after a delay, and it is shown in **Figure 6.6**.

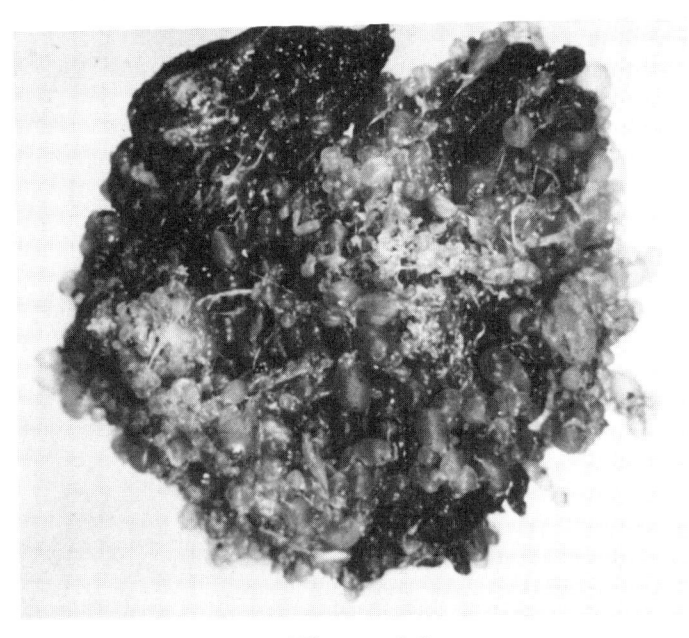

Figure 6.6

444. The findings indicate

    (A) normal placenta
    (B) retained segment of placenta
    (C) hydatidiform mole
    (D) invasive choriocarcinoma
    (E) chorioamnionitis

445. The patient should have which study in follow-up

    (A) CT of liver
    (B) pelvic sonography
    (C) endometrial biopsy
    (D) human chorionic gonadotrophin (hCG) measurement
    (E) D and C (dilatation and curettage)

446. The patient should be advised to

   (A) undergo immediate total abdominal hysterectomy
   (B) avoid pregnancy
   (C) undergo monthly checkups with pap smears
   (D) undergo tubal ligation
   (E) begin chemotherapy

ANSWERS AND TUTORIAL ON ITEMS 444-446

The answers are: **444-C; 445-D; 446-B**.

The specimen shown here is that of the patient's placenta and it represents a hydatidiform mole. To determine whether this represents an invasive mole, one of the earlier stages of the malignant placental tumors that include choriocarcinoma and other trophoblastic neoplasms, human chorionic gonadotrophin (hCG) assay after pregnancy is helpful. The patient should be advised to avoid pregnancy, since pregnancy itself will give an hCG elevation, and that would lose the utility of this hCG marker as a proxy for recurrent tumor. Under the circumstances of recurrence, the patient would be advised to undergo hysterectomy as the possibility that this mole might have been invasive would be sustained by evidence of its recurrence.

Items 447-449

A 34 year-old man who had lived 15 years in East Africa was found to have a renal mass on sonogram (**Figure 6.7A**) which was performed for suspected cholecystitis. CT scan confirms the presence of the mass (**Figure 6.7B**) and its location in the kidney.

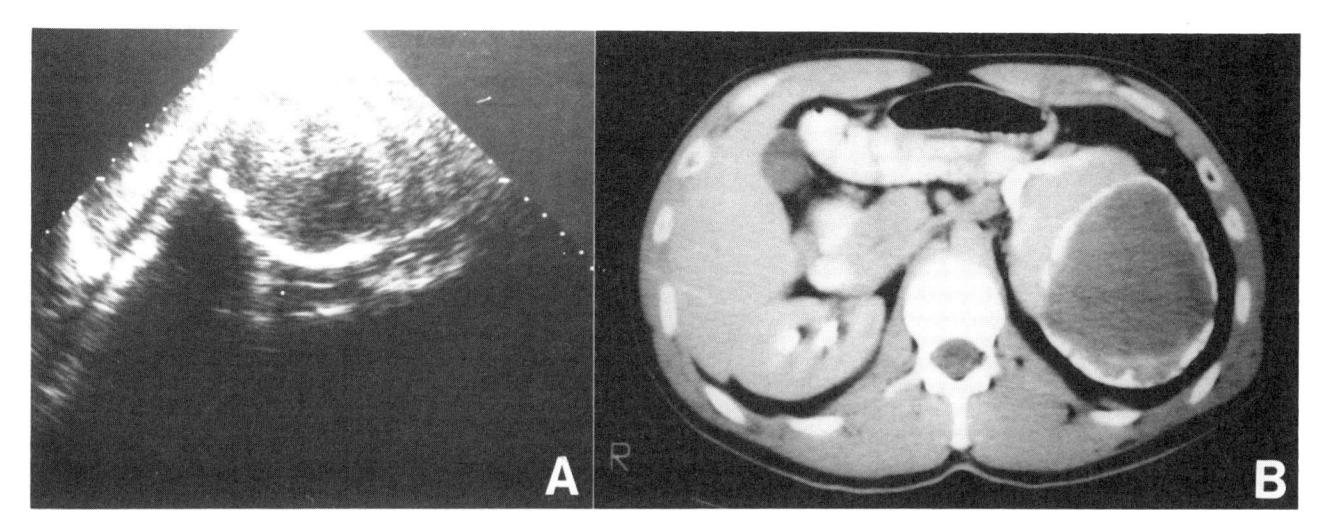

Figure 6.7

447. The cyst is likely to be of what origin?

    (A) polycystic kidney disease
    (B) *Echinococcus* cyst
    (C) medullary sponge kidney
    (D) hypernephroma with central necrosis
    (E) organizing hematoma

448. The chief concern in operative manipulation of this mass is

    (A) hemorrhage
    (B) spreading the tumor
    (C) spilling contents
    (D) vascular invasion
    (E) lymphatic drainage

449. A potential consequence of this mass' presence over an extended time includes each of the following **EXCEPT**:

   (A)   rupture
   (B)   anaphylaxis
   (C)   hypertension
   (D)   urinary stones
   (E)   bacteremia

ANSWERS AND TUTORIAL ON ITEMS 447-449

The answers are: **447-B; 448-C; 449-E**.

This patient presents with a renal mass that turns out to be an *Echinococcus* cyst. It was incidentally discovered, since it had caused him no symptoms, and the chief concern in the operative manipulation is to avoid spilling its contents. The reason to avoid this phenomenon is the probability of spreading the disease through daughter cysts from the scolices as well as anaphylaxis that may result from exposure to this antigenic material.

Items 450-452

A 52 year-old man had painless hematuria and a palpable flank mass on examination. Sonogram (**Figure 6.8A**) showed a mass with arteriogram (**Figure 6.8B**) and cavagram (**Figure 6.8C**) following this study and preceding the OR exploration (**Figure 6.8D**).

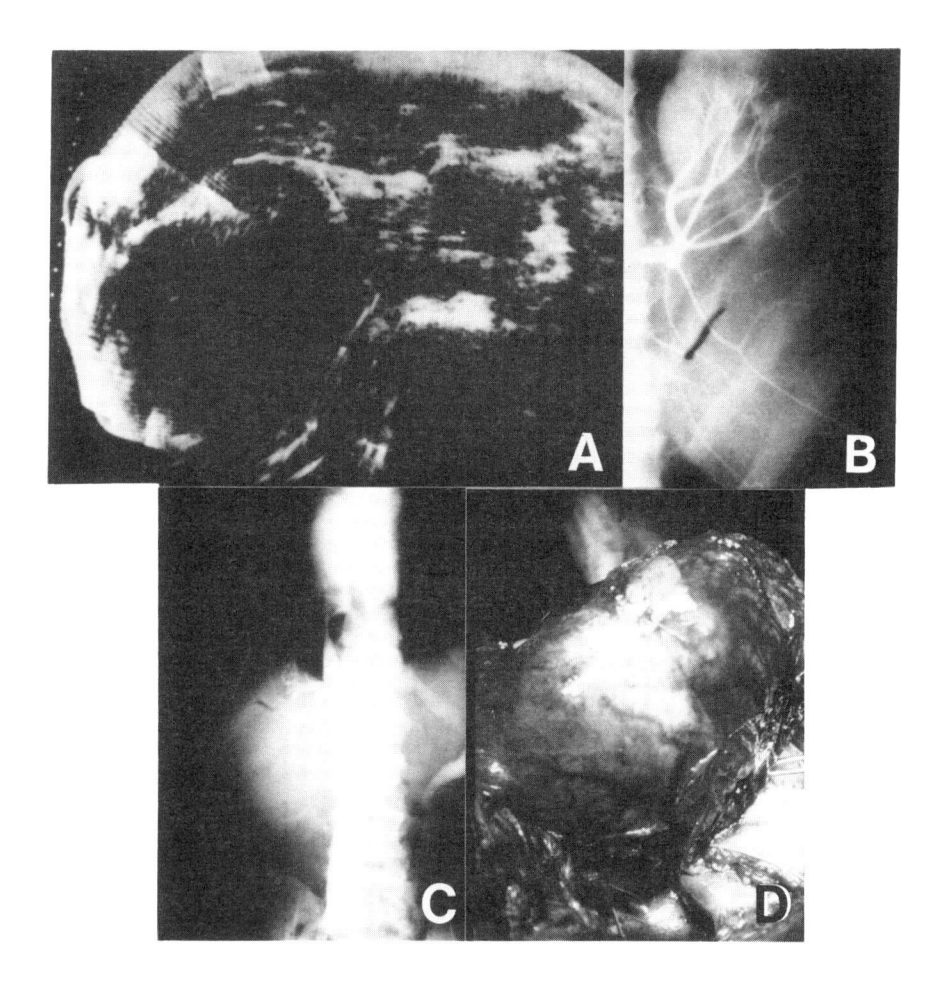

Figure 6.8

450. The importance of the vascular studies is to

 (A) plan subtotal nephrectomy
 (B) delineate Gerota's fascia for tumor bloc
 (C) reveal hepatic metastases
 (D) demonstrate intravenous extension
 (E) place venous occlusion-coil

451. The tumor in this case is most likely

    (A) renal cyst
    (B) Wilms' tumor
    (C) hypernephroma
    (D) metastatic
    (E) epidermoid

452. Early components of the operation will include each of the following steps **EXCEPT**:

    (A) low ligation of the ureter
    (B) arterial ligation
    (C) biopsy of the tumor mass
    (D) control of intravenous extension
    (E) *en bloc* dissection

ANSWERS AND TUTORIAL ON ITEMS 450-452

The answers are: **450-D; 451-C; 452-C**.

This patient has a large hypernephroma. The important components of this hypernephroma are seen on the cavagram with an intravenous extension. Should the kidney be removed and this tumor thrombus within the cava be persistent, not only could the tumor disseminate through this hematogenous means, but also the thrombus and tumor embolus itself can be a problem as can any pulmonary embolus. During the dissection of this tumor, early arterial ligation will help control bleeding and early control of the venous extension of the tumor will limit the spread of this tumor which will be dissected *en bloc*.

What will not take place is biopsy of this tumor mass. The biopsy would violate the "bloc", and the pattern of X-ray leaves little doubt as to the nature of this mass. The biopsy would not change treatment as far as the radical *en bloc* nephrectomy is concerned, and the definitive diagnosis will be obtained by histology of the resected specimen.

Items 453-456

(A) Undescended testis
(B) Torsion of testis
(C) Both
(D) Neither

453. testicular malignancy

454. infertility

455. acute emergency

456. operation by scrotal approach

ANSWERS AND TUTORIAL ON ITEMS 453-456

The answers are: **453-A; 454-C; 455-B; 456-D**.

An undescended testis is infertile, since the lower body temperature of the scrotum is necessary for spermatogenesis. The undescended testis, if left in its high inguinal position for a prolonged period, has successively higher risks of later associated malignancy. This malignant threat is not a component of torsion of the testis, which is an acute emergency presentation. If torsion of the testis results in infarction, sperm production may be reduced, but fertility should not be impaired unless both testes were involved. That is true also for the undescended testis, and infertility results from both conditions if it is bilateral. The operation for both conditions is carried out by a groin incision, as a scrotal approach should not be employed for most operations on the testis.

Items 457-461

(A) Intraductal papilloma
(B) Fibroadenoma
(C) Breast abscess
(D) Paget's disease
(E) Fibrocystic disease
(F) Bilateral inflammatory breast carcinoma
(G) Infiltrating intraductal adenocarcinoma
(H) Lobular *in situ* adenocarcinoma

457. A 16 year-old is found to have firm mobile nodules in both left upper and right lower breast quadrants.

458. The most common lethal condition of women in the prime of life.

459. A 28 year-old woman who has breast pain and fever with onset during her second month of nursing.

460. A benign condition that can give a bloody nipple discharge.

461. A scaly nipple rash associated with underlying malignancy requiring further investigation.

ANSWERS AND TUTORIAL ON ITEMS 457-461

The answers are: **457-B; 458-G; 459-C; 460-A; 461-D**.

The distinction of benign from malignant is the most important diagnostic feature of breast disease. Characteristic clinical patterns make the probability more or less likely in any given list of characteristics, but it is important to remember that breast cancer is not only the leading nonskin cancer in women, it is the overall most likely cause of death in women in the Western world in the prime of life. It is for that reason that cancer's early recognition should be distinguished from among the other benign breast problems that out-number it.

Dominant nodules are often the earliest presenting feature of breast cancer, but in a teenager, they most often represent a firm and rubbery kind of tumor known as fibroadenoma, particularly if multiple.

A bloody nipple discharge can be a presenting sign of cancer, but it is also characteristic of a benign condition known as intraductal papilloma from which it must be distinguished. One of the harbinger signs of breast cancer is a peculiar scaly nipple rash known as Paget's disease, and it is not so much a diagnosis as a mandatory indication for further investigation. In the context of lactation, a focal tender breast mass in the region of the areola is likely to be a breast abscess. These benign conditions are treated differently from breast cancer; however, the most important step in that treatment is their differentiation to rule out a malignant tumor which may sometimes co-exist.

Items 462-466

(A) Fine needle aspiration
(B) Needle localization biopsy with specimen mammography
(C) Incision and drainage
(D) Excisional biopsy
(E) Quadrant subtotal mastectomy
(F) Total mastectomy
(G) Modified radical mastectomy
(H) Extended radical mastectomy
(I) Radiation therapy
(J) Anti-estrogen therapy
(K) Prosthetic breast reconstruction
(L) Combination chemotherapy

462. Treatment for non-palpable stippled calcification seen on screening mammogram.

463. Appropriate therapy for a 92 year-old woman with congestive heart failure found to have an ulcerating 6 cm left breast mass.

464. Appropriate outpatient management of a patient with bilateral upper outer quadrant breast nodularity with one nodule firmer and larger than the surrounding tissues.

465. The best adjunctive treatment to be used following modified radical mastectomy for estrogen receptor-negative, poorly differentiated Stage II carcinoma in a premenopausal woman.

466. The most frequent operation performed in the US in the last five years for treatment of Stage I breast cancer in premenopausal women also treated by radiation therapy.

ANSWERS AND TUTORIAL ON ITEMS 462-466

The answers are: **462-B; 463-F; 464-A; 465-L; 466-E**.

The invasive procedure for definitive diagnosis of breast cancer depends on whether the lesion is palpable or whether it is a screening finding on mammography. If not palpable, its precise targeting is difficult without radiographic assistance. Marking it with needle insertion with the assistance of mammography gives needle localization technique a chance to sample the very specific tissue identified as suspicious by mammography, and to confirm that it has been excised for biopsy with specimen mammography. In a woman who has findings in several fields of the breast that may resemble fibrocystic changes, but with one dominant nodule, invasive diagnosis is still required for that dominant nodule. Out-patient management would include fine needle aspiration of the suspicious component.

For the majority of women with Stage I carcinoma at premenopausal ages in the US, quadrant sub-total mastectomy is combined with lymph node sampling for staging and primary radiotherapy is administered with the breast conserving procedure. An alternative is mastectomy with immediate reconstruction, which is a somewhat more invasive undertaking. Neither condition results in a normal postoperative breast appearance, but in each instance women may look nearly normal in clothes. If the disease turns out to be Stage II, particularly if undifferentiated, adjunctive chemotherapy administered in combination drug regimens is recommended. For an elderly patient with compromised cardiac reserve, who presents with an enlarged ulcerating breast mass, the principle threat to life is the cardiac rather than the oncologic problem. Breast tumors in such individuals are frequently indolent, but can cause local disfiguring and socially unpleasant problems, and this morbidity can be reduced by what is referred to as "toilet mastectomy" which rids the principle problem related to the large breast tumor — namely, the ulceration and soilage. For the great majority of women with breast cancer; however, therapy is tailored toward that which gives the highest probability of prolonged disease-free survival, and secondarily to morbidity reduction related to the treatment, particularly the loss of the breast.

Items 467-471

    (A)   Femoral hernia
    (B)   Indirect inguinal hernia
    (C)   Direct inguinal hernia
    (D)   Umbilical hernia
    (E)   Para-esophageal hernia
    (F)   Incisional hernia
    (G)   Richter's hernia
    (H)   Sliding hiatal hernia

467. Medical treatment indicated.

468. No treatment is typically recommended.

469. An incarceration.

470. High potential for hemorrhage.

471. More common in girls than in boys.

ANSWERS AND TUTORIAL ON ITEMS 467-471

The answers are: **467-H; 468-D; 469-G; 470-E; 471-A**.

    A sliding hiatus hernia is treated medically, not so much treatment directed to the hernia as to minimize the damage that may occur with esophageal reflux. In contrast, the other hernia at the hiatus is the para-esophageal hernia, which has high potential for hemorrhage in entrapment of the richly vascularized gastric wall. The presence of a para-esophageal hernia is indication for operation. For the umbilical hernia, particularly in the infant and toddler stage in which it is most often seen, no treatment is typically recommended. Should umbilical hernia persist or recur later in life under circumstances of increased intra-abdominal pressure such as pregnancy, it may then become symptomatic, and this may indicate its repair. Of the hernias listed, the Richter's hernia is an incarceration of partial circumference of the bowel wall. Of the inguinal hernias, indirect inguinal hernia is the most common hernia in young girls, even more common in young boys. However, girls have femoral hernias more often than do boys, even though femoral hernias represents a minority fraction of the groin hernias for both genders.

Items 472-476

    (A)   IVP excretory urogram
    (B)   Voiding cystourethrogram
    (C)   Retrograde pyelography
    (D)   Renal perfusion scan
    (E)   Renal arteriogram
    (F)   Computed tomography (CT)
    (G)   Ultrasound
    (H)   KUB flat plate (kidney, urinary bladder)

472. Sometimes treats as well as diagnoses ureteral calculi.

473. First screening test for kidney stones.

474. Indicated in male trauma patient with blood at external urethral meatus.

475. May be an early sign of acute rejection episode.

476. May define extension of hypernephroma and be useful in reducing its size pre-operatively.

ANSWERS AND TUTORIAL ON ITEMS 472-476

The answers are: **472-A; 473-H; 474-B; 475-D; 476-E**.

    Excretory urography uses an intravenous bolus of contrast material that acts as an osmotic diuretic. Not only does it opacify the urinary collecting system, the osmotic effect causes a diuresis and dilatation proximal to the obstructing lesion that might be diagnosed by IVP and simultaneously may clear by the dilatation and peristalsis of diuresis facilitating stone passage. A first screening test for presence of kidney stones is the flat plate abdominal film known as KUB, for encompassing the region of the kidney and urinary bladder with the ureter in between. If there is an opaque stone (as the majority of calcium oxalate — the most frequent calculi — are, with the exception of urate stones) it is frequently visible in the urinary tract distribution if other extensive calcification or opacity such as barium does not obscure it.
    An IVP would not be the first study for a patient who has a drop of blood at the urethral meatus, in which disruption of the urethra or distal urinary tract outlet from bladder down would be more likely than a higher urinary tract lesion, and voiding cystourethrography would be recommended to define the area of potential disruption.
    Since rejection is an early vascular phenomenon and usually is accompanied by a rise in vascular resistance to perfusion, a renal perfusion scan is frequently the sensitive early indicator

of acute rejection episodes in a transplanted kidney. Renal arteriography is a very useful study in hypernephroma to define the extent and extension of the tumor and its frequent site of capsular or intravenous invasion. In addition, through the same arteriography catheter, an obstruction can be introduced into the artery through a spring coil with Dacron wool. This will shrink the size of the tumor when employed immediately pre-operatively and facilitate the resection.

Items 477-486

477. Each of the following constitutes a risk factor for breast cancer **EXCEPT**:

    (A) heredity
    (B) fibrocystic disease
    (C) nulliparity
    (D) prolonged breast feeding
    (E) prior breast cancer

478. Signs of breast cancer include each of the following **EXCEPT**:

    (A) bloody nipple discharge
    (B) skin dimpling
    (C) Paget's disease of the nipple
    (D) breast discomfort
    (E) unilateral nipple retraction

479. Which of the following cancers of bone is **LEAST** common?

    (A) primary osteosarcoma
    (B) breast carcinoma
    (C) lung carcinoma
    (D) prostate cancer
    (E) thyroid carcinoma

480. In a 36 year-old woman with a painless hard dominant breast lump, the next step should be

    (A) mammography of the lump
    (B) fine needle aspiration cytology
    (C) radiation therapy
    (D) radical mastectomy
    (E) bone scan

481. Which of the following breast lesions is typically benign?

    (A) cystosarcoma phylloides
    (B) comedocarcinoma
    (C) lobular carcinoma
    (D) medullary carcinoma
    (E) intraductal carcinoma

482. Mammography should be employed

    (A) annually for asymptomatic women over age 30
    (B) to screen other areas of the breast in an 18 year-old found to have a fibroadenoma
    (C) every 6 months in 30 year-old women identified as high risk
    (D) to definitively characterize a dominant mass discovered on physical examination
    (E) no more frequently than annually in asymptomatic women 50 years of age or older

483. Stage I carcinoma of the breast is characterized by each of the following **EXCEPT**:

    (A) tumor size smaller than 2 cm
    (B) two or more axillary lymph nodes are positive
    (C) no distant metastases are present
    (D) five year survival is 85% or more
    (E) estrogen receptors may be positive or negative

484. Each of the following represents premalignant disease or a risk factor for breast cancer association **EXCEPT**:

    (A) proliferative fibrocystic disease
    (B) fibroadenoma
    (C) Paget's disease
    (D) lobular carcinoma *in situ*
    (E) atypical ductal hyperplasia

485. Estrogen receptor activity can be characterized by which of the following statements?

    (A) positive only in breast cancer
    (B) will react only in binding estrogen
    (C) is associated with a poor prognosis
    (D) is positive only in premenopausal patients
    (E) is an indication for adjunctive endocrine therapy

486. Current adjunctive therapy for a premenopausal 40 year-old woman following radical mastectomy with a 2.5 cm ductal carcinoma with 2 of 15 lymph nodes involved and an estrogen receptor negative tumor includes

   (A) tamoxifen
   (B) cytotoxic chemotherapy
   (C) androgens
   (D) oophorectomy
   (E) pituitary irradiation

ANSWERS AND TUTORIALS ON ITEMS 477-486

The answers are: 477-D; 478-D; 479-A; 480-B; 481-A; 482-E; 483-B; 484-B; 485-E; 486-B.

477. Earlier prior breast cancer in the patient or first order female relatives increases the risk of breast cancer as does prolonged estrogen stimulation as is seen with nulliparity. Dysplastic changes in fibrocystic disease may be precursors of neoplasia. Prolonged breast feeding interrupts estrogen stimulation and is actually protective against the development of breast cancer.

478. Pain is often associated with inflammatory conditions, and if the neoplastic change causes a secondary inflammatory component, breast discomfort may be associated with breast cancer, but it is not typically due to it. Retraction or a specific scaly rash of the nipple (Paget's disease) or a bloody nipple discharge along with a dimpling or depression of the skin are serious signs of breast cancer, often associated with a painless lump.

479. Primary bone cancer is the least likely of those cancers listed. Metastatic disease to the bone is much more frequent, and breast and lung cancers are very frequent carcinomas metastatic to bone. Both thyroid carcinoma and prostatic carcinoma have a high predilection for bony metastasis.

480. Mammography is not indicated for a mass that requires cytologic or histologic identification, so mammography of a suspicious lump will not change the indication for its biopsy. Neither radiotherapy nor mastectomy are appropriate until diagnostic confirmation of carcinoma is confirmed either by cytology or subsequent biopsy at which point therapeutic options can be discussed, and bone scan would only be appropriate as a prediction of metastatic disease which still would require primary breast cancer diagnosis and treatment.

481. Despite the misleading name, cystosarcoma phylloides is an atypical rapidly growing variant of fibroadenoma. It is almost always benign, with lymphatic metastases very uncommon and malignancy occurring in less that 10%.

482. A clinically discovered mass requires invasive cytologic or histologic diagnosis and not mammography. Other parts of the breast might be examined to determine therapy, but not for an 18 year-old with a suspected fibroadenoma. Even for patients with high risk, repeated mammography at short intervals, particularly at younger ages, should be avoided. The current recommendation is for asymptomatic women to be screened annually after age 50.

483. Positive axillary lymph nodes represent breast cancer at Stage II disease which decreases survival at five years from 85% to 66%. Stage I disease has no distant metastases, and a small primary tumor size, in which estrogen receptors may or may not be positive.

484. Despite its name, many authors regard lobular carcinoma *in situ* as a premalignant finding rather than true carcinoma, and Paget's disease is often a harbinger of breast cancer. Atypical hyperplasia and florid fibrocystic disease are both associated with excess breast cancer risk, but fibroadenoma is not associated with such risks.

485. Estrogen receptors are found in breast tissue, and other tissues such as colon cancers or colon tissue in either gender. They react with ligand-binders in addition to estrogen, such as antestrogens, e.g., tamoxifen. They are not only associated with premenopausal patients, and confer a better prognosis in those patients largely because they do constitute an additional indication for an adjunctive therapy with endocrine treatment.

486. The patient described has Stage II carcinoma which requires adjunctive therapy in current clinical opinion. The alternative treatments represent endocrine therapy that would be recommended if estrogen receptors were positive, but negative estrogen receptors in this younger woman suggest a poorer prognosis that would be best treated by adjunctive chemotherapy.

Items 487-496

487. Which of the following statements are **NOT** true regarding prostate carcinoma in a 95 year-old man?

    (A) presence of prostate carcinoma is 95% likely in the prostate of any 95 year-old American man
    (B) treatment should be designed to prevent the spread of the disease
    (C) it is associated with an elevated prostate specific antigen
    (D) it typically follows an indolent course
    (E) management is by observation

488. Which of the following processes involving the kidneys does **NOT** produce hypertension?

    (A) polycystic kidney disease
    (B) renovascular stenosis
    (C) glomerulonephritis
    (D) nephrectomy
    (E) coarctation of the aorta

489. An agitated 28 year-old man comes to the emergency room stating he is having another episode of ureteral colic, having previously passed urate stones on several occasions. He states he is allergic to intravenous pyelogram (IVP) contrast. He demands Demerol. His urinalysis is unremarkable. The most likely diagnosis is

    (A) urate stones
    (B) von Munchausen's syndrome
    (C) narcotic addiction
    (D) IVP contrast hypersensitivity
    (E) a malpractice litigant baiting the clinician

490. A 14 year-old boy enters the emergency room with bright red blood at the urethral meatus. He is not forthcoming with any history, and his midstream urinalysis is unremarkable as are other preliminary laboratory studies. A likely diagnosis might be

    (A) prostatitis
    (B) instrumentation
    (C) epididymitis
    (D) mumps
    (E) syphilis

491. A newborn male has bilateral flank masses and sonographically confirmed hydroureter. The most likely diagnosis is

   (A)   uretero-vesicle stenosis
   (B)   bilateral suppurative pyelonephritis
   (C)   primary hydronephrosis
   (D)   infantile prostatism
   (E)   urinary bladder atresia

492. A patient with normal blood pressure, blood counts, and blood chemistry is noted to have an opaque calcium calculus in both kidneys incidentally described on a routine chest X-ray. On an IVP, multiple diffuse cysts were seen in both kidneys. Repeat examination is again normal and the patient denies symptoms. A likely diagnosis is

   (A)   polycystic kidney disease
   (B)   von Hippel-Lindow syndrome
   (C)   medullary sponge kidney
   (D)   miliary biogenic renal metastases
   (E)   septic arterial emboli from infected cardiac valve vegetations

493. Arteriography may be employed in the defining of the extent of the blood supply of hypernephroma but has what additional principal advantage?

   (A)   it would rule out operation by demonstration of hepatic metastases
   (B)   it would determine unresectability for cure by demonstration of renal venous tumor extension
   (C)   it can be used to facilitate operation by occluding the principal and collateral blood supply to the tumor
   (D)   it may involve demonstration of portal venous tumor invasion
   (E)   chemotherapeutic transcatheter infusion is delivered direct to the tumor

494. Each of the following treatments is acceptable in managing benign prostatic hypertrophy **EXCEPT**:

   (A)   proscar (Fenastamide)
   (B)   transurethral resection
   (C)   suprapubic prostatectomy
   (D)   perineal prostatectomy with interstitial radiation therapy
   (E)   transrectal biopsy and observation

495. A 56 year-old woman with chronic fatigue has mild anemia and eosinophilia on blood count, and occult microscopic hematuria on clean catheterized urinalysis. A sonogram ordered to check her pancreas suggests a left renal mass. A likely diagnosis is

    (A) glomerulonephritis
    (B) renal carbuncle
    (C) hypernephroma
    (D) squamous cell carcinoma of the renal pelvis
    (E) stag-horn calculus

496. Newer techniques alternative to pyelolithotomy include all the following **EXCEPT**:

    (A) basketing the stone for retrieval by ureteral catheter
    (B) ECSW lithotripsy
    (C) chemically dissolving calcium oxalate stones by infusion into the kidney
    (D) pulverizing the stone by laser or shock energy introduced through ureteral catheterization
    (E) laparoscopic minimally invasive nephrolithotomy

ANSWERS AND TUTORIALS ON ITEMS 487-496

The answers are: **487-B; 488-D; 489-C; 490-B; 491-D; 492-C; 493-C; 494-D; 495-C; 496-C**.

487. It is inappropriate to do radical therapy to contain the threat of malignant spread in a tumor of almost any kind in a 95 year-old patient, particularly prostate cancer. Since it is very likely to be present, and it is less likely to be causing problems because of its indolent behavior, observation would be adequate to see if there were symptoms related to it. It there were, treatment would be related to those symptoms, such as relief of urinary tract obstruction or bleeding.

488. Renovascular hypertension may occur with arterial stenosis or proximal narrowing as in coarctation, atherosclerosis or fibromuscular hyperplasia. Polycystic kidney and glomerulonephritis can also result in nephrogenic hypertension, since while the kidney is present it can give rise to renin which produces hypertension as an end result of its peptide activation sequence. If the kidney is absent, it not only does not excrete, it doesn't secrete either, so nephrectomy should not be associated with a hypertensive response.

489. With a well practiced story, patients who request narcotic often get it when the story cannot be corroborated, and urate stones would not be radio-opaque, and could not be demonstrated if IVP contrast were contraindicated. The urinalysis does not suggest hematuria, and his agitated state might suggest either psychic problems (and the story a component of the von Munchausen's syndrome) or narcotic withdrawal. IVP contrast hypersensitivity can be tested for, but not with results in the period of time during which he requires his alleged pain to be treated. Narcotics should be withheld until further confirmation of his alleged problem is corroborated. So as not to withhold information from him regarding your reasons for not complying, he should be told about the skepticism, not regarding his pain, but regarding his diagnosis which cannot be confirmed.

490. There is no evidence for urinary tract pathology beyond the urethra, and the clinical context is that often seen with manipulation and fear of consequences. Mumps would have acute orchitis and the inflammatory conditions of epididymitis or prostatitis are not likely to give a negative physical exam and blood work. This is not the presentation of chancre, either, so the patient should be invited to talk about his fears to the limit that he is willing to do so over a follow-up observation.

491. This syndrome is recognized to be a feature of newborn males, and it is embryologically derived in an obstructive uropathy also known as "posterior urethral valves." These paramesonephric (Müllerian) remnants give a high grade obstruction which causes reflux and hydronephrosis with massive megaureter. The syndrome should be reversible with relief of the urethral valves and decompression if the renal cortex has not been totally destroyed, but in the newborn there is a good deal of resiliency for recovery. It is likely that the hydroureter will require ureteral tapering and reimplantation at a later stage in the process. There is no early reason why any newborn should have suppurative pyelonephritis or embryologic reasons why atresia or stenosis at other sites should develop, and that is why the particular anatomic point of obstruction has been termed infantile prostatism.

492. Medullary sponge kidney is often a surprise finding on IVP in patients who are undertaking this test for some other indication. Sometimes the medullary cysts have calcific calculi, and that may indicate the study, but not usually for cause of ureteral colic, since the stones are not often released into the collecting system. The other options are not likely to be the underlying diagnosis in an asymptomatic patient, particularly those that deal with pyogenic inflammatory processes. Polycystic kidney has a different distribution of the cysts, which typically enlarge the kidneys much more and von Hippel-Lindow findings are associated with this syndrome beyond the presence of renal cysts, such as retinal findings and liver abnormalities.

493. Hypernephroma is one tumor that is better managed surgically following radiographic devascularization. A spring coil with thrombogenic material can be placed in the feeding vessels and reduces tumor bulk and vascularity encountered in subsequent operation. This is also a method for stopping hemorrhage in tumor or palliating patient by tumor reduction in metastatic sites. Arteriography would not reach the portal venous system and would not be used for identifying hypernephroma extensions to it which would be unlikely. Both identification of hepatic metastases, or intravascular extension into the renal vein would not contraindicate operation, since patients respond to tumor reduction in the former instance, and the patient can still be cured even with demonstrated presence of intravascular venous invasion.

494. Benign prostatic hypertrophy's management is principally designed to relieve urinary tract obstruction symptoms and also to rule out the presence of malignant prostate disease. If there is no obstruction, observation can be safely followed after biopsy confirmation in some age groups that no malignant prostate component is present. Open prostatectomy was the standard before wide-scale application of transurethral resection techniques, but now a new therapy has been made available in the form of an enzyme inhibitor that shrinks benign prostatic hypertrophy and may postpone or eliminate the requirement for operations designed to relieve obstruction. This tendency toward more benign and less invasive procedures for benign prostatic hypertrophy would preclude a radical perineal prostatectomy, and no interstitial radiation implant source would be required for the benign disease.

495. A complex of microscopic hematuria, eosinophilia and a renal mass strongly indicate hypernephroma. The patient is not the right age for glomerulonephritis, and squamous cell carcinoma is typically found only after prolonged resident renal calculus which is not suggested by the sonogram. Metastasis to the kidney would be more unlikely than the primary origin of this tumor in the kidney given the triad of the findings.

496. Although lesser invasive procedures have been developed for kidney stone removal, most have involved cystoscopic manipulation of ureteral catheters to retrieve stones or fragments or pulverizing the stone through extracorporeal shock wave lithotripsy or direct contact with the stone through the ureteral approach. As yet, no available chemical dissolves the calcific stone without causing damage to the surrounding tissue that would preclude its use.

CHAPTER VII

NEUROSURGERY
PEDIATRIC SURGERY
ORTHOPEDIC SURGERY

Items 497-499

A 48 year-old man had fallen and struck his head 6 months earlier, and presented 3 months after injury with forgetfulness, astereognosis, and lateralizing signs. Operation revealed a collection of fluid described as "old engine oil".

497. The source of this fluid would be

    (A)   bridging veins
    (B)   middle cerebral artery
    (C)   arterial aneurysm
    (D)   middle meningeal artery
    (E)   meningeal tumor

498. The location of this fluid collection is

    (A)   inner table of the skull
    (B)   subdural
    (C)   epidural
    (D)   intracerebral
    (E)   arteriovenous malformation

499. Prognosis following operation should be

    (A)   nearly complete recovery
    (B)   10% 5 year survival
    (C)   stable neurologic deficit without progression
    (D)   50% 5 year survival
    (E)   probable recurrence within 2 years

ANSWERS AND TUTORIAL ON ITEMS 497-499

The answers are: **497-A; 498-B; 499-A**.

This patient has the classical clinical presentation of a subdural hematoma. The time course and the nature of the injury relate to the tear in the bridging veins that give rise to this collection of blood and the operative appearance of "old engine oil" confirm this as subdural hematoma. Following drainage of this collection, recovery should be nearly complete if there were no prior neurologic difficulties that gave rise to the fall in the first place.

Items 500-503

(A) Wilms' tumor
(B) Neuroblastoma
(C) Both
(D) Neither

500. the younger, from newborn to 2 years old, the higher the incidence

501. catecholamine secretion

502. combination chemotherapy effective

503. benign transformation with growth occasionally occurs

Items 504-507

(A) Meningioma
(B) Glioblastoma
(C) Both
(D) Neither

504. benign

505. rarely cured

506. intracerebral

507. encapsulated

ANSWERS AND TUTORIAL ON ITEMS 500-503

The answers are: **500-B; 501-B; 502-A; 503-B**.

Neuroblastoma is the commonest malignant extracranial tumor in children. The higher incidences are in the younger ages. In fact, many premature stillbirths can be found with the tumor, many more than are seen in incidence after live birth. This should lead to the inference that the tumor goes away with growth and development of the newborn. And, it rarely does. The very encouraging inference drawn from the high incidence of neuroblastoma in premature still births, the lower incidence in live births at term and the decreasing incidence with the child's age advancing toward two years of age and the very rare cases of maturation of the undifferentiated neuroblastoma toward the benign ganglioneuroma — all give a window into the potential reversal of carcinogenesis; however, this is not translated into very hopeful therapy for these tumors.

Surgical treatment is the mainstay for neuroblastoma resection. Screening for this tumor can include catecholamine secretion which is variably present, secreting different species of catecholamines depending on the stage and grade of the tumor at the child's age. After surgical treatment, however, the last bright hope for cure has passed, since highly aggressive therapy including combination chemotherapy has not been effective in contrast to Wilms' tumor where even subtotal resection has had prolonged survival with combination chemotherapy protocols used as adjunct to operation.

ANSWERS AND TUTORIAL ON ITEMS 504-507

The answers are: **504-A; 505-B; 506-B; 507-A**.

Meningiomas are tumors of the dura. Consequently they have compressed dura that may encapsulate them. They are benign, and although not always resectable, they have a high success rate for surgical resection depending on their location and size. They can even be re-operated on if there is recurrence after subtotal resection.

Glioblastomas, however, are not from dural origin but from glial origin and as such do not encapsulate as much as spread by finger-like projections in the brain parenchyma. Both because of their malignant dedifferentiation and because of their growth pattern, surgical cure is rare. Most palliative therapy would be directed toward decreasing intracranial pressure as the mass expands, but there is some strategic question as to whether that would extend to removing the craniectomy skull plate to allow continuous expansion of the tumor with potential complications of draining, sepsis and discomfort from cerebral protrusion through the cranium. Prolonging functional survival might include medication for cerebral edema and occasionally radiotherapy for a period of consciousness, and then a merciful coma when elevated intracranial pressure is not relieved by these measures treated in a closed cranium.

Items 508-511

(A) Epidural hematoma
(B) Subdural hematoma
(C) Both
(D) Neither

508. chronic

509. bridging veins

510. lucid interval

511. concussion

ANSWERS AND TUTORIAL ON ITEMS 508-511

The answers are: **508-B; 509-B; 510-A; 511-C**.

The principle difference between epidural hematoma and subdural hematoma besides their obvious anatomic location above or beneath the dura is that the former is from *arterial* bleeding accumulating very rapidly under arterial pressure, and the latter is from venous bleeding which originates from torn bridging *veins* with the corresponding venous pressure limiting the hematoma's rate of accumulation. This difference immediately suggests that subdural hematoma may be chronic and may even be diagnosed at some distance in time after the closed head injury during which it was sustained. Epidural hematoma is an emergency.

Both are most often accompanied by concussion, and both are injuries that typically come from deceleration blows on the head, although, particularly in older individuals, the trauma may be minimal enough to have been forgotten by the time a late subdural hematoma diagnosis is made. That is rarely the case with epidural hematoma which not only is associated with a concussion, but is often accompanied by skull fracture, and peculiarly the fracture through the temporal area that entraps the middle meningeal artery, one of the most frequent sources of arterial hemorrhage into the head subsequent to trauma to the skull. Because a concussion occurs at the time of the blow, but it clears readily, the patient may be normal in cerebral function for a period of time until arterial pressure has caused considerable collection of blood and the patient loses consciousness for a second time after this lucid interval.

Treatment of both types of bleeding into the cranium involve decompression and hemostasis, but the epidural is a true neurosurgical emergency that should be recognizable and treatable by most physicians with surgical experience because of the very short time interval from the second loss of consciousness to the likelihood of "coning" — herniation at the foramen compressing the brainstem which would stop the vegetative functions of respiration and control of heart rate.

Items 512-514

A 42 year-old man has recurrent headaches and nausea following resection of a brain tumor 2 years before. Arteriography (**Figure 7.1A**) showed a finding confirmed at operation (**Figure 7.1B**) with the removal of a lesion (**Figure 7.1C**).

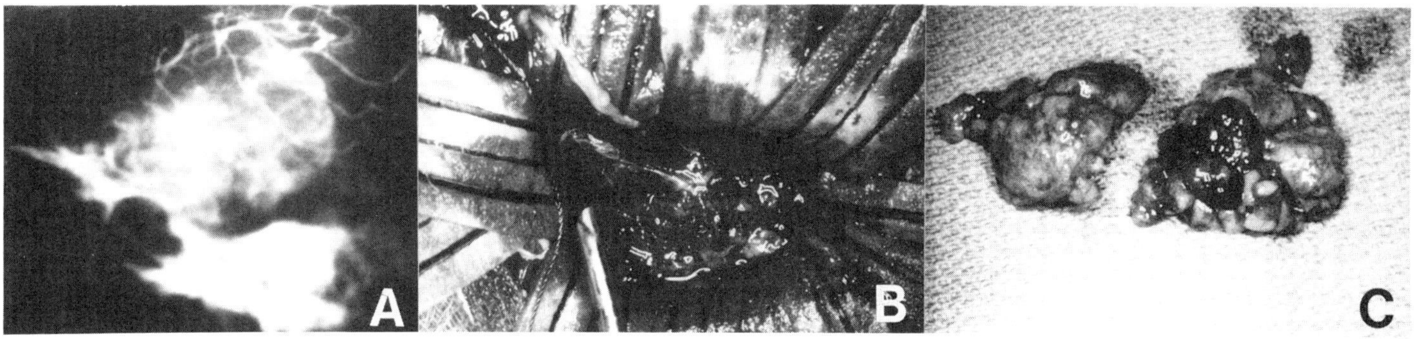

Figure 7.1

512. The nature of this mass is

    (A)   inflammatory
    (B)   metastatic
    (C)   dural in origin
    (D)   vascular in origin
    (E)   neuronal in origin

513. Prognosis for 5 year survival of incomplete resection of such a lesion is

    (A)   less than 5%
    (B)   10%
    (C)   25%
    (D)   50%
    (E)   greater than 75%

514. If recurrence appears, it would most likely be by

   (A)   hematogenous spread
   (B)   lymphatic metastases
   (C)   pulmonary nodules
   (D)   hepatic metastases
   (E)   local spread

ANSWERS AND TUTORIAL ON ITEMS 512-514

The answers are: **512-C; 513-E; 514-E**.

This patient has a 2 year course from the prior operation that he had for a brain tumor. Some brain tumors are much more rapidly growing than that, and this would likely rule out some of the most malignant of the brain tumors. That local resection is attempted again is also suggestive of the nature of this lesion which originates in the dura mater. This patient has a recurrent meningioma. Even incomplete resection of this lesion would likely give a prognosis of greater than 75% at five years. The recurrence of such a lesion is usually local rather than metastatic in some fashion, rarely if ever leaving the skull through hematogenous or lymphatic routes. Local recurrence should be treated by repeat operation as in this instance.

Items 515-523

515. Which of the following statements concerning papilledema is **NOT** true?

    (A) it results from intracranial obstruction of the retina's venous drainage
    (B) it is seen as a primary problem in diabetes mellitus
    (C) retinal hemorrhages and exudates are often associated
    (D) loss of venous pulsations is an early feature
    (E) increased intracranial pressure is the most frequent cause

516. Which of the following studies is contraindicated in a drowsy patient with papilledema whom one suspects of having acute closed head trauma?

    (A) carotid arteriography
    (B) lumbar puncture
    (C) CT scan
    (D) MRI
    (E) echoencephalograph

517. CT scan shows multiple solid 2 cm nodules in both cerebral hemispheres. This pattern is strongly suggestive of

    (A) glioblastoma multiforme
    (B) astrocytoma grade IV
    (C) multiple meningioma
    (D) metastases
    (E) pseudotumor

518. A 40 year-old man has developed ptosis of the left eyelid with the left pupil dilated in an eye that deviates laterally. He has no complaints of headache, dizziness or drowsiness, and this new finding has gradually worsened in four weeks. An arteriogram is ordered for evaluation with the clinical information of the request suggesting

    (A) meningioma, left frontal sulcus
    (B) left occipital arteriovenous malformation
    (C) pontine tumor
    (D) cerebellar aneurysm of basilar artery
    (E) left internal carotid aneurysm

519. Which of the following clinical signs is the most sensitive indicator of head injury from deceleration resulting in closed head trauma?

　　(A)　level of consciousness
　　(B)　blood pressure
　　(C)　pulse
　　(D)　cranial nerve function
　　(E)　deep tendon reflexes

520. A young man waiting for a bus was stabbed in the back and the his parcels were snatched. He fell without seeing his assailant, since he could not support himself upright because his right leg was powerless. On emergency room examination you find that he has a stab wound on the right side of the spine, but he has lost sensation in his left lower extremity. Other physical findings you would anticipate would include each of the following EXCEPT:

　　(A)　a loss of vibratory sensation on the right side
　　(B)　he has lost proprioception on the right side
　　(C)　he can distinguish heat from cold on the right side but not the left
　　(D)　the left lower extremity is hyperflexic
　　(E)　pinprick sensation is absent at the groin and left lower quadrant of the abdomen

521. Which of the following findings would be critically important information from skull X-rays or repeated examination and follow-up of the patient?

　　(A)　linear temporal skull fracture line
　　(B)　minimally depressed parietal skull fracture
　　(C)　midline suture separation of 1 mm
　　(D)　occipital linear skull fracture line
　　(E)　opacified left frontal sinus

522. Each of the following features of the Glasgow coma scale is true EXCEPT:

　　(A)　a Glasgow coma scale for an adult less than 7 is a good prognostic indicator
　　(B)　vocal response to the examiner at a measurement of 5 shows a well-oriented patient
　　(C)　motor response score 3 shows flexion indicating decorticate response
　　(D)　motor response at level of 2 shows extension indicating a decerebrate response
　　(E)　eye opening in response to pain is a positive response of 2

523. A 12 year-old boy was the catcher of a baseball game when he was struck in the lateral side of the head by the batter. He was knocked out, but revived a few minutes later and was comfortable, although complaining of a headache and scalp bruise in the emergency room, where he later became nauseated and drowsy. Appropriate management at this stage would be

(A) cerebral arteriogram
(B) discharge home in the care of his mother with a follow-up appointment in 72 hours
(C) hospitalization for observation following skull X-ray
(D) lumbar puncture
(E) outpatient CT scan scheduled for the following morning

ANSWERS AND TUTORIALS ON ITEMS 515-523

The answers are: **515-B; 516-B; 517-D; 518-E; 519-A; 520-D; 521-A; 522-A; 523-C**.

515. Increased intracranial pressure causes obstruction of venous return which first eliminates venous pulsations, leading to venous engorgement and papilledema which can then progress to hemorrhage and exudates in the retina. This process is an early sign of primary intracranial problems, and a patient with diabetes with these problems should have investigation of an intracranial pressure increase, since it is not associated primarily with diabetes.

516. A patient with an increased intracranial pressure as evidenced by papilledema has risk from lumbar puncture that can decompress the cerebrospinal fluid lower in the lumbar thecal space, and this may bring about a shift of the intracranial contents downward to cause herniation of the brain and compression of the medullary respiratory control centers. Consequently, no CSF should be withdrawn, nor should any loss be risked by leaking at a lumbar puncture site in a patient suspected of having acute intracranial pressure increase. Echoencephalography, CT and MRI scanning are imaging techniques that allow determinations of any shift in midline structures or identification of space occupying defects or swelling that may account for the intracranial pressure increase. Arteriography can show distortion of the vasculature which would allow an inference of the same information. Of the options, the lesser invasive studies would be preferred and lumbar puncture would be contraindicated.

517. Primary intracranial neoplasms may be invasive, and can become quite extensive, but are rarely multiple. That is true for both the lower grade neoplasms such as meningioma as well as high grade glioblastoma and astrocytoma. Pseudotumor is a clinical reflection of a variety of unrelated conditions that give rise to intracranial pressure increase from brain swelling, and would not show tumors, multiple or otherwise. The presence of multiple tumors in the substance of the cerebrum distributed bilaterally suggests metastatic cancer from an origin typically outside the head, most often spread by the hematogenous route.

518. Over half of the internal carotid aneurysms present with oculomotor nerve palsy, because of the adjacent structures' proximity. Without symptoms of increased intracranial pressure or dizziness, tumors, whether in the frontal sulcus or pons, would not be likely and do not explain the III nerve palsy, and the pontine tumor would be far more morbid in presentation. Vascular abnormalities in the occiput might give visual disturbances, more likely than cranial nerve dysfunction. Basilar artery aneurysms are rare, but in this instance would give symptoms of dizziness or imbalance. The internal carotid artery aneurysm on the left is the diagnosis strongly suggested.

519. In acute head injury, examination of the patient takes place after assessing the level of consciousness, since a conscious patient does not have disruption of the very sensitive indicator of cerebral function. Cushing response can be determined in a comatose patient by blood pressure and pulse, and tendon reflexes may help lateralize damage as might cranial nerve examination in a patient who does not have cerebral function. The level of consciousness is rather rapidly and readily assessed also making it a highly valuable indicator.

520. This patient has suffered a Brown-Séquard syndrome. Brown-Séquard described the clinical findings of this lesion which involve loss of motor innervation on the same side, and loss of sensation to pinprick and temperature on the opposite side of hemisection of the spinal cord. Both vibratory and proprioception sensation are also lost on the same side as the motor loss, since they are in the posterior column which is not crossed, similar to the motor innervation. The Brown-Séquard syndrome results from either a complete hemisection of the cord — in this case the right thoracic spine — or in compression of it or interference with its blood supply. There should be no change in motor reflexes in the left lower extremity which has intact motor innervation. (This clinical vignette, as are most of the others encountered in this book, is unfortunately not imaginary, but is a real story with recent history.)

521. Skull X-rays would be a low priority in the evaluation of patients with closed head trauma were it not for one critical area in which the skull fracture makes a clinical difference of urgent significance. Fractures in most areas of the skull would not be significant except in confirming the evidence of a severe blow to the head, and if not depressed considerably or displaced, no further surgical treatment of the fracture itself is indicated. That includes the parietal depressed skull fracture, and the very minimal suture line separation, and the occipital linear fracture. An opacified frontal sinus without antecedent history of sinusitis might suggest blood in the frontal sinus, but its presence there is not life threatening nor an indication of collateral critical injury. However, a linear fracture through the temporal bone runs a risk of disruption of the entrapped middle meningeal artery. Laceration of this artery would allow hemorrhage into the cranium under arterial blood pressure giving rise to an epidural hematoma which is an urgent threat to life. Subdural hematoma is under venous pressure, and accumulates more slowly and is frequently accommodated by patients over time, whereas epidural hematoma from the arterial hemorrhage that can be induced by this position of a linear skull fracture is life threatening.

522. The Glasgow coma scale is almost universally used for head injury patient evaluation. The three measured responses are to eye opening, motor response, and vocal response, with a score of 15 being an uninjured patient who is not ill. If six hours following injury, an adult has a Glasgow coma score less than 7, prognostic outlook is very poor. It is slightly better for such a low score in the pediatric age group.

523. Mechanism of injury in this patient in the clinical scenario are a worrisome combination suggesting a very significant head injury. What is described is a classic "lucid interval" whereby the patient suffers an immediate concussion and loss of consciousness, but recovers completely from that, only to begin deteriorating within a short period of time under observation. These findings suggest a rapid increase in intracranial pressure and that is often indicative of blood loss into the head. The position of the blow to the head could suggest a temporal or parietal location of the blow, and skull fracture that might have lacerated the entrapped middle meningeal artery, which can give rise to an epidural hematoma. The rapid accumulation of blood under arterial pressure often gives rise to the sequence of events described by this patient. Any option that would suggest discharge home, even under observation, would be inappropriate. The patient should have hospitalization for continuous observation as well as skull X-ray to evaluate the possibility of a linear fracture through the lateral skull. With increasing intracranial pressure, lumbar puncture is contraindicated, and CT scan might be appropriate, but certainly not as an outpatient and not the following day. Cerebral arteriography might be diagnostic, but there would be less invasive and more sensitive and specific studies with better reliability that could be achieved sooner. This patient has a serious problem that requires rapid evaluation and the probability of early intervention.

Items 524-526

You are called to evaluate a newborn infant who has had a low Apgar score, and still has inadequate color on weak crying 2 hours after birth, despite suctioning and Ambulatory Mechanical Breathing Unit (AMBU) ventilation. Chest X-rays AP (**Figure 7.2A**) and lateral (**Figure 7.2B**) are obtained and brought to you as you listen for breath sounds in the chest.

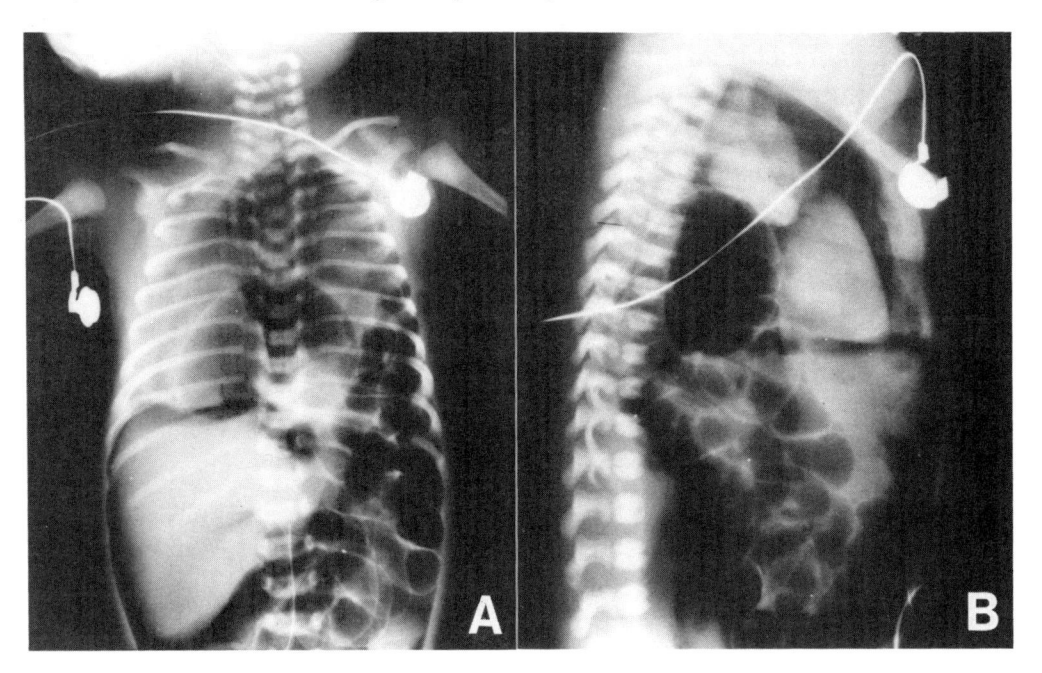

Figure 7.2

524. The likely diagnosis is

 (A) pulmonary sequestration
 (B) meconium aspiration
 (C) tracheoesophageal fistula
 (D) diaphragmatic hernia
 (E) tension pneumothorax

525. The next most likely complication to develop if this problem is untreated is

 (A) hemorrhage
 (B) perforation
 (C) hypoxic arrest
 (D) short gut syndrome
 (E) organizing pneumonia

526. The rate-limiting feature that most often determines survival in such infants is

    (A)   time to recognition of disease
    (B)   degree of pulmonary agenesis
    (C)   adequacy of antibiotic coverage
    (D)   capacitance of abdominal cavity
    (E)   oxygen toxicity

ANSWERS AND TUTORIAL ON ITEMS 524-526

The answers are: **524-D; 525-C; 526-B**.

The chest X-rays show a newborn with a congenital diaphragmatic hernia (of Bochdalek). A large proportion of the abdominal viscera is present in the chest through the incomplete separation of the pleural and peritoneal cavities by the congenital diaphragmatic defect. The presence of the bowel in the chest decreases the ability to ventilate. Even with suctioning, positive pressure ventilation, and intubation the patient has not yet become pink and well-oxygenated. Because of the persistent hypoxia, hypoxic arrest is a likely outcome. Because the defect is large, incarceration of the abdominal viscera within the chest is not likely. Although it is true that the viscera that have become resident in the chest have "lost domain" and the peritoneal capacitance may be decreased, the rate-limiting feature of diaphragmatic hernia is the concomitant failure of pulmonary development. The degree of pulmonary agenesis is often the feature that determines survival in such infants in whom the abdominal viscera are returned to the abdomen by several surgical techniques and the diaphragmatic hernia is repaired. But the adequacy of the lungs to maintain oxygenated blood in the newborn is more a function of the pulmonary immaturity, and sometimes this may require extrapulmonary oxygenation such as with extracorporeal membrane oxygenator use.

Items 527-530

    (A) Gastroschisis
    (B) Omphalocele
    (C) Both
    (D) Neither

527. peritoneal sac

528. postoperative respiratory insufficiency

529. staged repair

530. worse prognosis

ANSWERS AND TUTORIAL ON ITEMS 527-530

The answers are: **527-B; 528-C; 529-C; 530-A**.

    Omphalocele is a congenital defect in which the midline abdomen has a defect in which viscera are protruding in a peritoneal sac. The sac may be ruptured, either at birth or thereafter, but the bowel has been covered for at least the period of time up to diagnosis. Gastroschisis is also a midline upper abdominal defect, but does not have a sac lining, and the bowel is therefore often desiccated from exposure or contaminated, with inflammation and edema sometime to the point of devitalization.
    Since the portion of the gut that has been outside the abdominal cavity has not been accommodated during the period of intrauterine growth, there is no room for it in that there is no potential space that it has left behind in migrating outside the abdominal wall, since it did not develop inside the confines of that wall. For that reason, it must be returned gradually into the abdominal cavity which must expand to accommodate it. This is frequently done with prosthetic mesh material which is constricted in the form of a "chimney" to contain and preserve the bowel in a large prosthetic ventral hernia as gradual progressive staged procedures plicate more of this prosthesis and return more of the viscera to intra-abdominal position. If this were done rapidly, the diaphragm would be pushed up with respiratory insufficiency resulting, which remains a problem for both conditions. Because of the better state of the viscera at the time of the repair if the sac remains intact and protective for the omphalocele, gastroschisis has a worse prognosis than does omphalocele and the outlook for accomplishing the reduction of viable bowel into the abdominal cavity is worse. Once repair has been accomplished, prognosis is good for both conditions.

Items 531-537

531. The delivery room calls to report a newborn has been delivered with a protruding upper midline abdominal mass. You find that it is darkened, matted, stiff and dried without evidence of covering lining. The most likely diagnosis is

   (A) exstrophy of the bladder
   (B) omphalocele
   (C) eventration
   (D) gastroschisis
   (E) prune belly

532. Tracheoesophageal fistula is a congenital defect with several forms. The most common of these is

   (A) atresia of the trachea with a proximal segment of the esophagus connected to the distal tracheal stump
   (B) atresia of the esophagus with proximal and distal esophageal stumps adjacent to a normal trachea without fistula
   (C) esophageal atresia with a blind proximal pouch and a distal esophageal stump fistula connection to the trachea
   (D) atresia of the esophagus with both ends of the esophagus fistulized at different points to the trachea
   (E) tracheoesophageal fistula without atresia of either esophagus or trachea (H-type)

533. Which of the following statements is true regarding pyloric stenosis?

   (A) genders are equally affected
   (B) it is more common in Caucasians than Blacks
   (C) bilious projectile vomiting is characteristic
   (D) metabolic acidosis is a complication
   (E) its most common onset is 24 months of age

534. Wilms' tumor is a malignant renal tumor about which of the following statements only one is true?

   (A) if the tumor extends through the capsule of the kidney, survival is less than 50% following therapy
   (B) combination chemotherapy is a treatment recommended for nearly all patients as an adjunct to surgery
   (C) bilateral renal involvement is incurable
   (D) there are no recognized patterns of associated congenital anomalies
   (E) the tumor is not radiosensitive

535. Which of the following statements is true for the infant with persistent jaundice?

 (A) biliary atresia occurs before birth from intrauterine infection with hepatitis B
 (B) Australia antigen is invariably present with variable results to tests or the antibody against it
 (C) toxoplasmosis is frequently associated with intrahepatic biliary atresia
 (D) ultrasonography is most helpful in distinguishing surgically correctable biliary atresia from other forms of persistent jaundice
 (E) percutaneous external biliary drainage and refeeding bile into the upper GI tract through a tube is known as the Kasai procedure

536. Which of the following statements about pediatric neuroblastoma is true?

 (A) survival, compared stage for stage, is much better than for patients with Wilms' tumor
 (B) the older the patient is at diagnosis, stage for stage, the better the prognosis
 (C) patients with osseous metastases have a 50% complete response rate to combined radiation and chemotherapy
 (D) remarkable improvements in treatment success rate for advanced stage disease have progressed rapidly in the past decade from poor prognosis to better than even chance of survival
 (E) rarely it may be seen to mature with the growth of the infant, passing through neuroblastoma to ganglioneuroma.

537. Hirschsprung's disease is a colonic defect in children that results from

 (A) a bowel atresia acquired following birth
 (B) an infectious disease
 (C) a segment of colon that cannot relax, constituting a functional bowel obstruction
 (D) absence of parasympathetic innervation in the dilated megacolon
 (E) a rectum that appears normal but is devoid of parasympathetic ganglion cells in the myenteric plexus on submucosal biopsy

ANSWERS AND TUTORIALS ON ITEMS 531-537

The answers are: **531-D; 532-C; 533-B; 534-B; 535-D; 536-E; 537-E.**

531. This is a serious congenital abnormality and the outcome is determined by the condition of the viscera protruding from the abdomen at the time of treatment. Both gastroschisis and omphalocele have a protrusion, the former above and the latter at the umbilicus; however, the omphalocele is covered with a peritoneal sac and the bowel is typically in better condition because it is not as exposed as the stomach and the other matted viscera typically are in gastroschisis. Prune belly is a disorder of the abdominal musculature, and exstrophy of the bladder is a mucosal extrusion above the pubis at the lower rather than the upper end of the abdominal midline. Eventration refers to a chronic condition of the diaphragm not used in the context of this newborn congenital anomaly.

The viscera must be returned to an abdomen that has not accommodated them, after care is exercised regarding the vitality of the bowel and blood supply to it. This usually involves creating a new extraperitoneal environment for the bowel before gradually reducing it in steps into the abdominal cavity.

532. Esophageal atresia with a proximal blind pouch and a distal tracheoesophageal fistula (TEF) connecting the trachea to the distal atretic end of the esophagus occurs in nearly 90% of instances. The much more readily envisioned and discussed H-type fistula between both nonatretic esophagus and trachea (analogous to the acquired tracheoesophageal fistula in adults) is only 5% of the total of TEFs. Atresia of the trachea would be hypothetical, since such an infant would not survive to diagnosis. It is the esophageal atresia with or without connection to the trachea that has survivability since breathing is not totally impaired.

533. There is a peculiar age, gender, and race predilection to this disease with an etiology that is unknown but with some apparent mixture of hereditary and environmental factors. The majority of patients are Caucasian males, with the most common onset in infancy from two weeks to two months. Projectile vomiting is characteristic, but it is nonbilious because of the obstruction at the level of the pylorus. The vomiting, however, does give rise to a complication that is metabolic alkalosis rather than acidosis because of the vomiting of gastric acid.

534. Wilms' tumor is one of the earliest examples which suggests adjunctive systemic chemotherapy and tumor reduction could be employed with successful outcome for even advanced disease. Even when metastases to liver and lungs are present or when the tumor is bilateral, patients still have better than 50% survival prognosis. A whole list of associated congenital anomalies have been described in association with Wilms' tumor. The tumor is radiosensitive, and advanced stages of the disease are treated with radiotherapy, but there is a high complication rate to this treatment when high doses are employed with children. Wilms' tumor appears to be an ideal arena for the multidisciplinary treatment of cancer with a successful outcome in the majority that would not be intuitively obvious given the extent of the disease in some instances that respond to combined treatment.

535. Persistent jaundice must be differentiated in the newborn as in the adult from causes that are hepatocellular or those related to the collecting system. Toxoplasmosis may be a source of hepatitis as may hepatitis-B virus, but neither is invariably associated with biliary collecting abnormalities. In fact, biliary atresia and jaundice do not occur *in utero*, but are acquired after birth with no proven association with any one of a number of candidates for transmittable disease. The Kasai procedure is an internal drainage of a filleted liver porta into the upper GI tract, and does not involve percutaneous bile drainage. To distinguish surgically correctable biliary tract atresia from that which occurs too proximal in the liver or that which is due to hepatocellular disease (both of which would require replacement by means of liver transplantation) ultrasonography is most helpful, since dilated ducts and the presence or absence of a gall bladder may be visible for anatomic definition of the level of the atresia.

536. Neuroblastoma is the most common solid tumor in newborns, and one that has yielded least to the combined assault of surgery, radiation, and chemotherapy. The classic neuroblastoma may rarely be seen to mature with the growth of the infant, passing through neuroblastoma to ganglioneuroma, a benign encapsulated tumor that can be excised and the patient cured despite earlier biopsy diagnosis of the same tumor at birth confirming undifferentiated neuroblastoma. There have been no remarkable improvements in survival, which is uniformly worse than that seen with Wilms' tumor and gets worse with advancing age of the patient at diagnosis. With the possible exception of massive chemotherapy and radiation that ablates both tumor and bone marrow with marrow transplant rescue as an experiment, treatment has been based in frustration with the failures of regimens that had worked so well with Wilms' tumor. A rare insight into tumor biology is the occasional evidence of tumor maturation under the influence of some factors not clearly understood but certainly not entirely due to the pressures of therapy. Neuroblastoma is a tumor awaiting an infusion of new information before it can be managed.

537. The megacolon of Hirschsprung's disease is an acquired phenomenon, but the congenital defect is an absence of parasympathetic ganglia in the myenteric and submucosal plexus of the nondilated component, usually the rectum. This is not an atresia, but does constitute a functional bowel obstruction, since it cannot propel. The dilated portion of the colon is hypertrophic, responding normally to normal innervation propelling against this functional obstruction. There are many associations, including Down's syndrome, enterocolitis, and an overwhelming predominance in male infants and those affected with strong family history. Although it mimics some abnormalities seen with Chagas' disease, this congenital Hirschsprung's disease is not infectious.

Items 538-540

A 72 year-old woman had osteoarthritis with left knee more severely involved than the right. After prolonged consideration while maintained on steroid therapy, she underwent operation on her left knee depicted.

538. Each of the following adjuncts to operation is indicated **EXCEPT**:

    (A)   antibiotic prophylaxis
    (B)   corticosteroid replacement
    (C)   thromboembolism prophylaxis
    (D)   prolonged bed rest
    (E)   physical therapy

539. A likely subsequent operation will be to

    (A)   remove the hardware from left knee
    (B)   drain infected hematoma
    (C)   release contracture of left hip
    (D)   place vena cava filter
    (E)   replace right knee

540. The most serious debilitating surgical complication for which extraordinary preventive measures are directed is

    (A)   deep venous thrombosis
    (B)   atelectasis
    (C)   joint infection
    (D)   three unit blood loss
    (E)   decubital ulcers

ANSWERS AND TUTORIAL ON ITEMS 538-540

The answers are: **538-D; 539-E; 540-C.**

    This patient is undergoing a total knee prosthetic replacement. Because of her prolonged steroid therapy she will surely require steroid treatment as coverage for her operation. Antibiotic prophylaxis and thromboembolism prevention are certainly components of her therapy, but prolonged bedrest is not. The reason is that most patients who have this operation are going to be severely debilitated by a prolonged period of bedrest and must be mobilized early. This is also part of the physical therapy of the prosthetic knee replacement. It is likely that she will undergo subsequent replacement of the opposite knee, which will become even more burdensome to her when the newly rehabilitated function of the operated knee is apparent. It is highly unlikely that she will develop a joint infection, for which extraordinary means are expended to prevent this very serious debilitating surgical complication.

Items 541-544

      (A)   Proximal fibula
      (B)   Proximal tibia
      (C)   Both
      (D)   Neither

541. associated with treatment of compartment syndromes

542. healing fracture requires more than three months without weight bearing

543. bone graft donor site

544. internal fixation for alignment

ANSWERS AND TUTORIAL ON ITEMS 541-544

The answers are: **541-A; 542-B; 543-A; 544-D**.

The proximal fibula is expendable. It does not contribute significantly to the stability of the knee as it does indispensably to stability of the ankle at the lateral malleolus. In fact, the proximal fibula is sometimes taken as a donor bone graft for implantation elsewhere, and is excised and simply discarded in a patient who has a compartment syndrome, as in the case of postischemia reperfusion or crush injury of the legs.

In contrast, the proximal tibia is not only the articular surface of the knee, but also the sole source of support to weight bearing on the leg. Alignment to take this weight bearing stress is important, but that is typically achieved through external fixation and a prolonged period of healing with immobilization excluding weight bearing for three months or more to prevent malunion. The proximal fibula is not fixed at all, and the tibia generally aligns without the need for internal fixation.

Items 545-548

    (A) Bone fracture
    (B) Ligament sprain
    (C) Both
    (D) Neither

545. trimalleolar fracture

546. more common in children

547. very often requires casting

548. screw fixation

ANSWERS AND TUTORIAL ON ITEMS 545-548

The answers are: **545-C; 546-A; 547-C; 548-A**.

With a proportionate amount of joint trauma, the child would be more likely to break bone and the adult tear ligaments as a general rule. The ligament itself may avulse the bone in some instances, particularly around joints with considerable leverage such as the ankle, knee or elbow. When the ligament holds and bone is avulsed, frequently screw fixation can fix the bone which has failed before the ligament did. It is not the case that a fracture is more serious than a ligament injury, and both very often require immobilization in a cast. The mechanics of a blow that would disrupt the mortise of the ankle to give a trimalleolar fracture has likely done ligamentous injury as well, and this ankle will likely be significantly damaged and may be unstable despite closed and/or open fixation.

Items 549-552

    (A)   Femur fracture in child
    (B)   Femur fracture in elderly
    (C)   Both
    (D)   Neither

549. hip contracture common

550. internal fixation is the rule

551. immobilization advisable

552. traction is a preferred treatment

ANSWERS AND TUTORIAL ON ITEMS 549-552

The answers are: **549-B; 550-B; 551-A; 552-A**.

As anyone who has tried to restrain a child into an unwanted position knows, the young are very limber and nimble. Immobilization of a limb in which a fracture lies between joints rarely results in any contracture of those joints in a child; whereas, it would be common in an older individual to have contracture. This is particularly true in the hip which contracts in flexion. Immobilization, then, is advisable for the femur fracture in the child either by the preferred traction method or by some form of hip spica immobilization. This would be a disservice in the older person who has such disability secondary to immobilization that early ambulation is the rule, which is why internal fixation becomes the first choice of treatment for femur fracture in the adult.

Items 553-562

553. Each of the following maxims of management of extremity fractures is true **EXCEPT**:

    (A) avoid mobility in the upper extremity, preventing nonunion for a solid fusion
    (B) open fractures are contaminated wounds and treated as potential osteomyelitis
    (C) avoid conversion of any closed fracture to an open fracture by immobilization and splinting to minimize soft tissue damage
    (D) orthopedic management is a second order priority following shock resuscitation
    (E) avoid mobility in lower extremity fractures to prevent nonunion and achieve a solid fusion

554. Which is the ultimate criterion of successful outcome from orthopedic management?

    (A) correct anatomic alignment on X-ray
    (B) no visible deformity on clinical exam
    (C) adequate function of the part post injury
    (D) primary healing without evidence of callus
    (E) the shortest possible duration of the treatment course

555. Hematogenous osteomyelitis in patients with sickle cell anemia may uniquely be due to

    (A) *Staphylococcus aureus*
    (B) *E. coli*
    (C) *Hemophilus*
    (D) *Gonococcus*
    (E) *Salmonella*

556. A 9 year-old girl falls from her bicycle on her outstretched arm and is seen in the emergency room complaining of pain about the shoulder. The most likely diagnosis is

    (A) impaction fracture of the proximal humerus
    (B) Colles' fracture
    (C) acromioclavicular ligament tear
    (D) clavicle fracture
    (E) fracture of the radial head

557. "Clipping" in football is an illegal procedure incurring penalty on the part of the perpetrator. The injuries sustained by the one clipped resulting from force to the lateral aspect of the knee is likely to include each of the following **EXCEPT**:

   (A) hemarthrosis
   (B) tear of the medial collateral ligament
   (C) inter-trochanteric fracture
   (D) anterior cruciate ligament disruption
   (E) torn lateral meniscus

558. A middle-aged woman is knocked down and run over by a taxi, sustaining a crush of the right knee with open fracture with fragments of tibia protruding through the skin. Surgical management of this injury should include each of the following **EXCEPT**:

   (A) arteriography
   (B) open surgical debridement
   (C) copious irrigation with saline solution
   (D) prolonged systemic antibiotics
   (E) emergency total knee replacement

559. Which of the following fractures is **LEAST** clinically significant and can be treated without casting or immobilization?

   (A) fracture of the medial malleolus and deltoid ligament disruption of the ankle
   (B) fracture of the fibula at the lateral malleolus
   (C) trimalleolar fracture
   (D) fracture of the head of the fibula
   (E) fracture of the calcaneus

560. Which of the following statements regarding femur fractures in preschool children is true?

   (A) if perfect alignment of fracture fragments with anatomic continuity seen on X-ray takes place in the treatment alignment, the fractured limb is likely to grow longer than the normal opposite side
   (B) internal fixation is generally necessary
   (C) an intramedullary rod accelerates recovery for earlier rehabilitation
   (D) hip contracture is a significant problem with plaster spica immobilization
   (E) management with traction is inappropriate in young children

561. Which of the following statements is true for fractures that occur in children?

(A) the epiphyseal growth plate and its junction are infrequently the site of fracture involvement since this area of the bone is more flexible than bone in mid-shaft which is where most fractures in children occur
(B) a "greenstick" fracture is a transverse fracture breaking through the cortex on both sides of a long bone
(C) in a fracture through the cortex on one side of a long bone in children with the opposite cortex intact, during fracture reduction of an angulated deformity the opposite cortex should actually be broken to complete the fracture
(D) appropriate casting involves immobilizing the joint above, but not necessarily below the fracture site
(E) because they are growing, children's bones knit more slowly than those of adults who do not have the more widespread demand on calcium deposition

562. An elderly patient experiences a fall in circumstances not recalled by the patient or witnessed by others. The patient was brought by ambulance to the emergency room because he could not get up, when found by a daughter. Even with assistance, weight-bearing on the left is impossible. In the emergency room, raising the sheet to expose the feet you note that the left leg is shortened and externally rotated with the foot flat in bed on its lateral surface with the toes pointing to the patient's left. On X-ray you expect to find

(A) an impacted spiral fracture of the mid-femoral shaft
(B) an inter-trochanteric fracture
(C) a fracture separation of the pelvic symphysis
(D) impaction of the femoral head through the fractured acetabulum (arthrokatadysis)
(E) a pathologic fracture

ANSWERS AND TUTORIALS ON ITEMS 553-562

The answers are: **553-A; 554-C; 555-E; 556-D; 557-C; 558-E; 559-D; 560-A; 561-C; 562-B.**

553. The *mobility* of the upper extremity is crucial for normal function. Therefore, nonunion in fracture healing is preferable to a fused joint. The patient who cannot get his hand to his mouth or manipulate it in maneuvers of daily care cannot take care of himself, and is permanently disabled requiring attendants. If a fracture through a joint appears such that fusion is likely, the joint should be excised rather than to have it fused in a position of nonfunction. The *stability* of the lower extremities is functionally crucial. Here any mobility that might be a result of midshaft nonunion is a severe disability. Stable fusion is required for weight-bearing, and if that should require fusion of a joint, that is preferable to excess mobility that cannot be weight-bearing.

Open fractures are contaminated and potentially infected, and the handling of bony fractures should avoid further damage to soft tissue including conversion to an open fracture. So long as it achieves the desirable functional result, closed fixation is less of a risk than open fixation with the additional potential contamination.

554. Anatomy is less important than physiology as a criterion of end results. If a hand looks very abnormal, but functions as a hand, it is preferable to a cosmetically pleasing but nonfunctional result. Radiographic alignment in perfect anatomic reduction is often not desirable to achieve long term optimum function, particularly in younger patients. Remodeling of bone will take the place of precise alignment so long as function is not impaired. All healing occurs by bone callus, so that minimum callus may not be preferable (e.g., in a femur fracture where a large callus is desirable for strength). A short course that achieves a dysfunctional result is almost never to be preferred over a protracted process with functional end result.

555. Of all forms of hematogenous primary osteomyelitis to originate in the metaphysis of growing bones, *Staphylococcus aureus* is the most common cause. However, unique to sickle cell patients is an unusual osteomyelitis due to *Salmonella*. Young children with ear infections may have *Hemophilus* and sexually active patients may have arthritis based in *Gonococcus*. The most common etiologic organism in all patients would be *Staphylococcus* and the one unique to sickle cell anemia patients is *Salmonella*. This clinical fact is significant because treatment is different predicated upon these findings.

556. Clavicle fractures are common in all age groups, but particularly in children, and result from the mechanism of injury as described. When the force of the fall is transmitted up the arm to the clavicle, that strut is the only connection of the upper extremity to the trunk, and can fracture with the stress. The clavicle is a membranous bone and heals very readily in nearly all instances when immobilized with a figure-of-eight immobilization. Colles' fracture and radial head fracture could both result from this trauma but neither would give rise to the discomfort around the shoulder. Acromio-clavicular (A-C) ligament injuries would not be likely in this age group, but this is a possible site of disruption in older patients, but not typically with this mechanism of stress from a fall on an outstretched arm as much as direct trauma to the shoulder.

557. Ligamentous injury in the knee can be worse in outcome than fracture of bone. Remember that stability is an important function of the lower extremity, and ligamentous disruption can lead to excess mobility and a loss of stability. When force is applied to the lateral aspect of the knee, soft tissue stretching occurs on the medial side, and the medial collateral ligaments may be the first to go. With further deformity, the anterior cruciate ligament is frequently torn, and with it meniscus tears occur. This is know as the "terrible triad of O'Donaghue" and may end at least an athletic career if the knee cannot be relied upon for stability in being "planted" for forceful maneuver. Hemarthrosis is nearly inevitable with the tearing of ligaments and their blood supply. The force at the knee should not give rise to femoral fracture, at least not at the level of the hip where fracture site is so much more common in older patients who begin to demineralize.

558. The crush injury sustained in a joint such as the knee has high likelihood of neurovascular injury as well. Physical exam is important, but arteriography can identify intimal disruption and partial separation of the artery even if minimal pulses are felt from collateral or other sources distally. Removal of the debris by sharp dissection and extensive irrigation are indicated as an emergency, and therapeutic levels of antibiotics are indicated. It is contraindicated to implant any foreign body in this degree of contamination, and it is uncertain whether the patient would need this form of prosthesis later. If the long-term result is a healing in fusion of the knee, recall that stability is the main function of the lower extremity and this may be more appropriate for the patient in terms of weight-bearing than an artificial knee would be, which would be very difficult to assess with the traumatic disruption of the joint early on after injury.

Any attempt at reconstruction with implantation of prosthesis soon after the injury would result in a nonunion at the traumatic bone disruption with a risk of osteomyelitis and potentially a pseudarthrosis at the site of infection. It is conceivable that the patient would have a fused knee and a functional pseudoarthrosis below the knee which might imitate in functional result that which could be achieved with a much later attempt at total knee replacement.

559. The purpose of the fibula in the lower extremity is joint stabilization at the ankle and secure ligamentous connections. The fibula contributes very little to stability at the knee, and is not weight-bearing in its upper proximal extension. In fact, the head of the fibula can be excised and frequently is for either bone grafting or for relief of compartment syndromes, without functional consequence. Therefore, a patient who has a fracture of the proximal fibula may be treated with minor analgesics and could even be given some weight-bearing support so as to minimize discomfort at the fracture site, but will not be concerned with stability of the lower extremity, since weight-bearing is intact as it is aligned through the intact tibia. Each of the fractures at the ankle and foot are significant, since they disrupt the anchoring position of important ligaments that hold the ankle mortis. None of them are treated without fixation in plaster immobilization and some instances are treated with open fixation as well.

560. The femoral fracture would not require internal fixation in children, and an intramedullary rod would be particularly inappropriate, since it would align the bone fragments anatomically with even greater length if there was some distance between the fragments in opposition.

The young child is going to be growing, and the later disposition of that hardware that will shrink relative to the size of the child is another consideration. Rehabilitation is not speeded by open reduction or internal fixation, and children tolerate traction which is the preferred form of management. Some overlap is not only acceptable but desirable, since increased vascularity in the fractured limb is a response to injury that makes epiphyseal overgrowth on the involved side very likely, so that limb length would be discrepant with the injured limb being longer if perfect anatomic opposition were achieved by careful reduction. Limb length discrepancy would obviously lead to a limp or other consequences with spinal and pelvic alignment. Femur fractures in young children can be handled with traction or plaster spica immobilization, and in young children contracture at the hip is not a problem.

561. Are you surprised by this response? It is not often that a clinician is ready to fracture a bone in order to set it, but in this instance, angulation may be accentuated on the side of the cortical fracture, with overgrowth at the fracture site deviating the alignment of the bone to the opposite side. By disrupting the bone across both sides, alignment can be maintained during healing, while perfect alignment at the time of reduction may be followed by angulation because of the healing. Because the growth plate in children's bones is weaker, a distressingly large number of children's fractures disrupt the growth plate with many associated problems in growth that cannot be completely predicted or ameliorated and add another dimension to expected functional result following treatment. Both the joint above and below the fracture is immobilized. It may be helpful to remember that "ortho pedics" means "straight child".

562. Pathologic fracture is a fracture that occurs spontaneously or results from minimal trauma in a bone weakened by a metastatic or primary bone tumor. An elderly individual with osteoporosis already has the weakening, which is most remarkable for the significant public health problem for the elderly of hip fractures sustained in falls. The foreshortening and external rotation suggests inter-trochanteric hip fracture. A spiral fracture of the midshaft in the femur would be unlikely without extraordinary circumstances in the mechanism of injury, since the demineralized femoral neck would be a much weaker site for the stress to disrupt. The arthrokatadysis (Otto pelvis) is a highly unusual disorder that may arise from a number of circumstances besides the trauma that brought this patient to the emergency room, and it is likely that a blow sufficient to perforate the acetabulum would likely break the hip at the femoral head as well if not preferentially. A pelvic disruption is not a necessary component of the symptoms presented, and is much more uncommon than hip fracture. This scene is a very common clinical phenomenon happening nearly daily in many emergency rooms with the injury described being the most common among them.